YOUR SECRET MIND

YOUR SECRET MIND
Getting to Know and Living with Your Unconscious

Hans Steiner

with Rebecca Hall

Routledge
Taylor & Francis Group
LONDON AND NEW YORK

First published 2017 by Karnac Books Ltd.

2 Park Square, Milton Park, Abingdon, Oxfordshire OX14 4RN
52 Vanderbilt Avenue, New York, NY 10017

Routledge is an imprint of the Taylor & Francis Group, an informa business

First issued in hardback 2019

British Library Cataloguing in Publication Data

A C.I.P. for this book is available from the British Library

ISBN-13: 978-1-78220-495-4 (pbk)
ISBN-13: 978-0-367-32999-0 (hbk)

Typeset by Medlar Publishing Solutions Pvt Ltd, India

TO MY MENTORS

Two in spirit: Sigmund Freud, who taught me to follow my dreams; Ludwig Wittgenstein, who taught me to be critical, especially of Sigmund Freud.

Two in spirit and in body: Helfried Nolz, who taught me English, Bernard Shaw, Oscar Wilde, and pragmatism; and Irvin Yalom, who taught me to be my true self.

—Hans Steiner

CONTENTS

INTRODUCTION

What is this book?

Elisabeth Kübler-Ross once said: "Should you shield the canyons from the windstorms you would never see the true beauty of their carvings" (Welch, Winters, & Ross, 2009). What she meant to convey is the thought that all of us are affected by adversity, sooner or later. But as we are affected by it, it also brings out the unexpected, perhaps hidden strengths in us, the hidden beauty. Adding to this thought, Victor Hugo (1874) pointed out: "To put everything in balance is good, to put everything in harmony is better." So, even after we face our dark sides, we still face the task of putting everything together, into a harmonic whole. In this book, we will show how these two quotes are relevant to all of us today. In order to grasp ourselves in our entirety, we need to go deep. This book introduces the reader and student to the unconscious mind, the hidden treasures and dangers it holds. The book is based on a popular course that has been taught through Stanford University's Continuing Studies Program and to undergraduates in one form or another for the past twenty-five years. Most students (and I hope readers) will find this guided discovery of their own unconscious mind fascinating and enlightening.

Why is it important to study the unconscious?

Understanding your own unconscious will increase your self-knowledge, expand your creative potential, and improve your mental and, likely, physical health. First, studying your unconscious will allow you to get to know yourself better and ultimately live a happier, more fulfilling life. Second, this process will enable and augment your creative potential in all its forms, be it writing, painting, photography, or some other medium. Understanding and accessing your unconscious will help you to reenergize your creative pursuits and get beyond potential obstacles, such as writer's block or being frozen with inactivity. Finally, as you get to know yourself better, you will become aware of the reasons why you may find yourself in unsatisfying, hurtful, or even dangerous situations. After your third speeding ticket in six months or your second divorce, you may start to ask yourself, "Why does this keep happening to me?" If you are often asking yourself, "Why do I keep doing this, even though I know it does me no good?" then attending to the automatic, reflexive parts of your psychology might be helpful.

Exploring your unconscious is not a necessary condition for being a healthy human. However, when you find yourself coming up dry creatively or repeating unproductive or harmful habits, investigating your unconscious processes and motives, and ultimately understanding yourself more deeply, can be useful.

This complex enterprise may not work for everybody, but I (Hans Steiner, M.D.) am confident that it will work for many, having witnessed over twenty-five years' worth of personal insight and growth in my students, which by now number in the thousands, in addition to having witnessed the growth in my patients; my friends; and of course, myself.

Who are we?

Hans Steiner

I was born in Vienna, Austria and received my Doctor medicinae universalis (Dr. med. univ. = M.D.) from the medical faculty of the University of Vienna in 1972. I joined the medical faculty at Stanford in 1978 and have taught, researched, and provided clinical care in this setting since then. Currently, I am professor emeritus (active) of psychiatry and behavioral sciences, child psychiatry and human development at the Stanford University School of Medicine and guest professor at the

Medical University of Vienna. I am a founding member of The Pegasus Physician Writers at Stanford, a group of doctors who write creatively.

You can find out more details about me on my website (www.hanssteiner.com), where you can get a glimpse of my academic and creative life to date; on Wikipedia (http://en.wikipedia.org/wiki/Hans_Steiner); and on my Stanford website (https://med.stanford.edu/profiles/Hans_Steiner). These sites are interlinked and enable you to cross-reference.

My interest in the unconscious mind dates back to my high school days in Vienna. Our much beloved Professor Helfried Nolz, who taught us English and philosophy, having spent the years of World War II in England, loved to introduce us to English culture, show us the links between Austria and England, and challenge us with writings by George Bernard Shaw, Ludwig Wittgenstein, and of course, Sigmund Freud. One of our tasks was to select a book by Freud and write a detailed report on it. I chose *The Interpretation of Dreams* and became completely taken in by it. The idea that as we sleep, we produce poetic and at times chaotic images and stories, which might help us understand ourselves better, was fascinating to me—as was the idea that in practicing such an art, one combined literature, poetry, and doctoring. Best of all, one made a decent living, a fact that most impressed my parents. I wrote a very enthusiastic piece. In typical Nolz fashion, what I got back was a good grade, but also a further challenge: I was asked to describe what Wittgenstein thought of Freud. The two were contemporaries, and Wittgenstein on several occasions had shown his appreciation of psychiatry. I found a piece by him on Freud; to my surprise, he basically issued a grave warning: He thought Freud was a deeply original thinker, but in order to learn from him, one had to be very critical (Barrett, 1966).

I discussed all this with Professor Nolz. He was very pleased that I had not become engulfed by Freud's theories, but was at the ready to examine, reexamine, and then decide what I thought were the pieces most valuable in his writings; what held up under intense philosophical and empirical scrutiny; and what could be discarded. "Freud," he said, "was brilliant, but human. He, like you and I, made mistakes. And Wittgenstein saw that very early on." We decided that since Freud's writings, the fields of psychology, psychiatry, and neuroscience had moved on with alacrity, developing tools that Freud could not even imagine.

It is in this spirit that I approach this book, my classes, my research, and my patients. I wrestled with the ideas of Sigmund, whom I greatly admire, for many years. A great deal of my research seeks to examine his theories. In fact, my very first paper, written as a psychiatric resident, sets out an agenda for my professional life, which I have followed for many decades (Steiner, 1977). This book contains much of what I have learned, researched, and been taught by other colleagues. It contains some very basic, useful, and empirically supported facts from depth psychology, which allows everyone access to deeply hidden aspects of themselves—aspects that may be strengths or hindrances, guideposts into the future or reminders of past bad times. Going through the exercises in this book may help to heal hurts, regain momentum to step into a fuller life, and bring out hidden creativities, which have not been recognized to date.

The other strong motivator to get to know my own and other people's hidden mind was that ever since high school, I have written creatively and have much appreciated novels, novellas, and poetry. In fact, my German professor in high school, Hermann Mayer, had high hopes for me becoming a novelist. He was very disappointed when I announced I was going to medical school. He recovered quickly though, saying that "We need doctors who write well," giving me the inspiration to pursue creative writing, first in German, and now in English. As I have continued to write and teach many other creative writers, artists, photographers, actors, and stand-up comedians, I have increasingly appreciated how important it is to have facile access to the more hidden aspects of one's mind. Robert Frost once said that "If you do not surprise yourself as you write [and I would add draw, paint, act, photograph, dance, etc.] why should the reader be surprised?" And it is true, sometimes as I write a poem or a story, a line or a paragraph springs forward that seems almost as if written by someone else. Writing without such moments to me now seems flat, journalistic, pedantic. You have to learn to let these underground streams of emotion and memories come up like a well and suffuse the story. This is not too different for the other medias of art, where as I have learned, a similar process pushes the artist in an unexpected direction—the actor into a role that he (or she, of course, but for simplicity we will let "he" or "she" apply to both) had not quite anticipated. And as you allow your unconscious to bubble to the fore in this fertilization process, would it not be nice to at least have an idea where it is going to take you, which elements will emerge, which emotions suffuse the art, whatever it may be? We will include a lot about the unconscious default network, which houses these emotionally linked surprises, in the following chapters.

In my creative writing in English, I have edited a volume of poetry, memoirs, and short stories by The Pegasus Physician Writers at Stanford, *On Becoming and Being a Doctor*. I have also published a psychiatric literary essay on the psychology and psychopathology of Lisbeth Salander, "If Lisbeth Salander Were Real," in an edited volume called *The Psychology of the Girl with the Dragon Tattoo* (Robyn Rosenberg and Shannon O'Neill, editors). Most recently, I have published two short stories in *The Intima: A Journal of Narrative Medicine*, describing the medical practice of a child psychiatrist working in a hospital setting ("Talking in Toys") and an important step in my acculturation to America ("The Cat Doctor").

I am continuing work on a collection of interlocked short stories, *Peripeteia: Tipping and Turning Points from the Mental Edge of Medicine*, which approaches the practice of developmental psychiatry from a literary perspective and shows how central psychiatry is to medicine. A second collection of longer stories about the unfolding of four patients' lives over the course of twenty to thirty years after initial treatment is entitled *Stepping into the River*. Both should be available within the next two years. Working on these books, I was inspired by Irvin Yalom, M.D., a much-treasured mentor and friend, who has been incredibly supportive and generous with his time. He of course is a psychiatrist who has most successfully modeled the reciprocal benefits brought from writing to medicine and vice versa. I was very happy to celebrate his achievements in a special invited paper, a traditional German "Laudatio," published in English in 2012. He is also one of the founding members, along with me and two others, of The Pegasus Physician Writers at Stanford, a group started in 2008 and now 100 members strong. We support our young colleagues in becoming the best physicians and writers they can be. We all believe that being a doctor overlaps with being a writer in significant ways. Writing makes us better doctors and keeps helping us to follow a calling which sometimes seems too hard to bear. (More information about the group can be found on the web at www.pegasusphysicians.com.)

Having had a dual career as an academic physician and writer, I am no stranger to publishing and editing, because that is one of the key demands in that role. As an academic, I have written more than 500 papers, abstracts, and book chapters. I have written and edited eleven textbooks (these titles can be viewed on my Stanford website and in the "Books by Dr. Steiner" tab on my website). My research and clinical practice are based on developmental approaches to psychopathology, which emphasize the conjoint study of normative and nonnormative phenomena and the complex interaction of biological, psychological, and social variables in the etiology, pathogenesis, diagnosis, and treatment of mental disorders. From this perspective, I approach the complex topic of the human unconscious as a source of creativity, wellness, personal improvement, and a potential receptacle of obstacles to healthy development. What I have learned though, as I have pursued these two tracks in all these years, is that my hidden mind is a sine qua non for creative writing, but not for the typical expositional nonfiction that one writes as a researcher. In fact, the two forms of writing are in some competitive relationship, so that when one is in the foreground, the other one recedes. In the past eight years I have found that I am more drawn—again—to creative writing, and although I have much to learn on that front, I am willing to pursue this form of human expression to the fullest. My hidden mind has given me permission and support to do that.

Rebecca Hall

I graduated from Stanford University in 2007 with a bachelor of arts in human biology, a concentration in abnormal and delinquent psychology, and a minor in Spanish language. I first met Dr. Steiner when I was a student in one of his classes during my sophomore year. I was then awarded an HB-REX internship from Stanford University to work in his research laboratory, where I learned about the various elements of academic research, from gathering and analyzing data to writing up the manuscript for publication. While I enjoyed the research process in general, I always looked forward to sitting down and writing up our findings.

After graduating, I began to focus more and more on writing and editing, though not yet full-time. I also started working as Dr. Steiner's teaching assistant for his Stanford Continuing Studies Course, "Your Secret Mind: Getting in Touch and Living with Your Unconscious." Each year I listened to his lectures about the material that you are about to read, and I watched student after student uncover pieces of themselves that they didn't know (or had forgotten) were there. I have greatly enjoyed getting to know these students each year and witnessing their growth. Perhaps because I am particularly drawn to writing myself,

I am always especially impressed by the insights that students are able to achieve about their unconscious mind through expressive writing.

After a few years as the teaching assistant, I was approached by Dr. Steiner about helping him with this book. At first, I was hesitant—more out of self-doubt than a lack of interest. Though I had heard him give these lectures countless times and I had worked on several journal articles by that point, I didn't know if I had the writing skills to do this project justice. However, Dr. Steiner was persistent, so I decided to give it a shot. Once I started writing, I knew that I had found my career.

I now work full-time as a freelance writer and editor, specializing primarily in the psychiatric and behavioral sciences and in translating scientific information for the general public. I have earned coauthorship on eight journal articles and ten psychiatric textbook chapters, and I have edited several additional publications. I am a coauthor and assistant content editor of the book *Treating Adolescents, 2nd Edition* (Hans Steiner, editor); the editor of *The Anti-Depressant Book* (Jacob Towery); the assistant content editor of *Handbook of Developmental Psychiatry* (Hans Steiner, editor); and the assistant content editor of *Eating Disorders* (Hans Steiner and Martine Flament, editors).

I also write creatively. My nonfiction stories have been featured at "Doctors and Patients: What We Learn from Each Other," a Pegasus Physician Writers at Stanford event; the 32nd annual "In Celebration of the Muse," a showcase of female authors; and in *Wildfire*, a digital magazine.

For more information, please visit my website (rebeccahall.net).

How this book achieves our goals

In this book, I (Hans Steiner, M.D.) will teach you how to utilize five channels of access to your unconscious mind. These channels are memes, slips, art preferences, expressive writings, and dreams. Each will be discussed in detail in Chapters Four to Seven. I will approach the task of teaching you how to access your unconscious by drawing on your entire human potential, creative and otherwise. I will appeal to your aesthetic sense and your appreciation of art, poetry, and beauty in all its manifestations, encouraging introspection and reflection. As humans are historical beings, I will invite you to remember your experiential development and explore how you came to where you are today. I will try to engage you in being creative, at the very least through expressive writing exercises, but also through activities such as photography, painting, and acting, as all these pursuits encourage you to manifest latent aspects of yourself that you might not normally be thinking about on a daily basis.

The theoretical roots for this book are found in "depth psychology," that is, the branches of psychology based on the theory that human behavior cannot necessarily be read only at face value, but can be an expression of underlying motives, past experiences and trauma, and adaptive stances which are no longer useful. In order to understand why people do things, you have to inquire within. These psychologies, which deliberately go beneath the surface, include the following: 1) Freudian psychodynamics, the theory that states that human behavior is the result of an interplay between intrapsychic and interpersonal factors, bringing conflicts and difficulties to a conscious work space to understand and consider options, and tailoring outcomes to more adaptive possibilities; 2) existentialism, which states that humans are free to make choices regarding their lives that shape their experiences in significant ways; 3) developmental psychology, which states that human existence is driven by internal positive forces that propel us towards adaptive health, that dysfunction can impede development, and that after symptom reduction it is important to reestablish the natural trend towards healthy change; and finally, 4) constructivist realism, which states that reality is not an objective Kantian *Ding an sich*, but an emergent state generated in the interpersonal dialectic between individuals. In this exchange, they alternatively state what they assume to be a socially agreed upon state of affairs and an intra-individual interpretation of what facts are, which of them are important and meaningful. Reality is assembled, not simply given. Nowhere is this as evident as when we approach a piece of art. I would argue that most great pieces of art are ambiguous. Although two people may stand in front of the same canvas—the same stimuli are presented to them and enter their brain—the interpretation of what the art means can differ greatly. Eric Kandel (2012), the Nobel Prize winning psychiatrist, has described the neuroscience underlying this process. What he has shown is that we all construct our realities based on our own experiences, beliefs, and attitudes. Art is a kind of mirror to us. We will use this process liberally in this book.

The theory that underlies this model is a combination of constructivist hermeneutics (we generate realities by interpreting what we see and hear) and the idea that humans have a direct access to reality transmitted through all senses, which requires no interpretation, but simply is. This toggling back and forth between what we intuitively know to be true and the reconstruction of how we came to believe that—the presence/hermeneutic dialectic—is at the core of the highest human capacities (Ricoeur, 1970). It is this ability that we will show you how to recognize and exploit to your advantage. It is this dialectic that is applied in the depth psychological therapies, where such an exploration takes place in the confines of a supremely private, confidential, and carefully managed therapeutic alliance.

It is of course also true that not all reality is subject to such profound processes of interpretation. There are simple forms we all can readily agree on, such as stop signs, directions on the freeway, or a user's manual for a computer. This kind of information is readily taken in and used in the way it is usually meant to function.

Another quick caveat though: In this course and book, we will not assess, diagnose, or treat. We will teach you the tools that overlap with psychiatry and psychology, but these tools can never replace medical diagnosis, psychological testing, or treatment interventions. These tools may, however, make it apparent to you that you might need such help. In my experience over the past decades, about 1–2 percent of students in my classes became aware of some psychiatric issue that they needed to take care of, as they were studying themselves with our methods. On the other hand, it also has become clear that students that had past or present experiences with psychotherapy were quite adept in completing these exercises, and excelled in producing most interesting results. This of course makes complete sense to me. Thus, this is a book that can be used as an auxiliary tool for those who are in treatment and are seeking to accelerate and solidify their progress. Another cautionary note is in order: In my experience, the students and patients who have most benefited from this approach are the ones that in a recent article, a meta-analysis by Jonathan Shedler (2010), have been found to benefit most from so-called psychodynamic treatment. Individuals that struggle more with neuro-psychiatric syndromes tend not to engage well, or have essentially been absent from my classes. Again, that makes sense to me as a clinician. Psychiatry has matured to the point where we do not expect that one treatment approach fits all. Brain injuries, intellectual disabilities, autism, and schizophrenia, to name a few causes, need other interventions which hold out much more of a promise to help and heal. In my textbooks, I have grouped disorders accordingly, but nowadays any sophisticated practitioner of the mental health sciences would agree with what I say (Steiner, 2011; Steiner with Hall, 2015).

I use the time-honored medical method of case-based teaching: you are invited to study a case in depth, and I suggest that case be you, yourself. If for some reason you do not want to use yourself in this process, this is of course okay. Maybe you have a willing friend or partner who would not mind serving as your case of study. But in my many years of teaching, I have found that studying yourself is usually the most productive way to proceed. I counterbalance your deep but idiosyncratic fund of knowledge with empirical, scientific, and clinically agreed-upon facts and will try to help you as best I can to embed your profile into a larger pool of people who have in fact taken these tests—usually thousands—by using the standardized ways of basic psychometric testing.

The introductory chapters (Chapters One to Three) bring you closer to the state of the art in the field of mental health. Chapter Three especially gets you close to the most important source of information regarding your secret mind: you, yourself. By completing a set of standardized screening tests which I have used in my clinic, laboratory, and field research extensively, you will get to know the sides of you that will in fact help you enter these exercises, or hinder you, as you are trying to do so. These tests require some but not a lot of familiarity with psychology and testing, but most of the students in my classes have put them to good use and comprehend their meaning.

Chapters Four to Seven use an empirical base to develop exercises that bring you directly into your unconscious. I use case material, art, and writing samples from famous artists and previous students who have given permission for us to do so.

First, I discuss the use of memes in understanding the unconscious. Memes, a term introduced in the 1970s by Richard Dawkins, are units of cultural information, such as a practice or idea, that is transmitted verbally or by repeated action from one mind to another. Examples include thoughts, ideas, theories, practices, habits, songs, dances, and moods. A well-known example of a meme is Winston Churchill's saying, "If you are going through hell, keep going." Nowadays, memes have acquired a somewhat different meaning on the internet. We are sticking to the original description. I also discuss parapraxes, which are errors in speech, memory, or physical action that are thought to reveal a repressed motive, such as "Freudian slips." Keeping track of these slips is usually difficult, and your partner or friends can catch them long before you do, but they can reveal information about the unconscious. Sigmund Freud dedicated a whole book to them (1901b).

Next, I discuss the concept of objective correlative, a term introduced by T. S. Eliot in his essay, "Hamlet and His Problems." Objective correlative is the artistic and literary technique of using symbols to evoke a particular emotion in the viewer or reader. As a result, upon viewing the piece of art or reading the text, the reader/viewer experiences the emotion that the artist was trying to impart. In the first chapter, I use a hermeneutic process of analysis—a method of interpreting human behavior, thoughts, and creative works—to analyze the psychology of the famous painter, Rene Magritte, and the viewer, or reader. In Chapter Five I discuss how art analysis and the hermeneutic process can aid you in accessing your own unconscious mind.

In Chapter Six, I discuss the use of expressive writing and narrative diaries in getting to know the unconscious. In this technique, you are asked to write for thirty minutes, undisturbed and unedited, about a positive or negative event. I show you how to use this stream of consciousness to access and understand unconscious processes. The technique has been studied for many years in psychology, mostly by James Pennebaker from the University of Texas at Austin. He has repeatedly shown the beneficial health effects of this practice. We are using a more recent, refined method to study your writings, closer to depth psychology, as developed by Wilma Bucci and Bernard Maskit.

Finally, in Chapter Seven, I discuss dream analysis. I have kept this exercise for last, because what I have learned over the years is that this is perhaps the most difficult one to achieve in class and with students who are working on their own. By leaving it for last, I also apply the knowledge from my classes that most students make more and more significant inroads into their secret minds as they do all the exercises. Thus, one reaps the benefits from all the previous chapters. I encourage you to keep track of your dreams in a dream diary, and I guide you through the analysis of psychologically significant dreams. Not all dreams are meaningful in a psychological way, but some can be used to reveal hidden aspects of oneself. My exercises help you to develop methods to distinguish meaningless dreams from significant ones, and I will teach you the most efficient ways of recording and analyzing dreams.

I will often use examples from my own repertoire to demonstrate each technique. This is not done out of a belief that my work is superior to others, but because, quite simply, it is free to reproduce. I can also be reasonably sure of the authenticity of these contributions. Throughout the book, discussions and examples will periodically alternate between genders.

Disclaimer

In the past years of teaching this class, I have learned not only to outline what this book will bring to you, but also to emphasize what this book (or class) is not. Above, I have tried to distinguish our book and course from clinical interventions. In addition, this is not a neuroscience book, although, as mentioned before, it will utilize the insights of neuroscience to lead you to interesting tools and analyses of the results of the five channels of access—memes, slips, art preferences, expressive writings, and dreams. You will not be able to obtain continuing medical education credit or credit for licensure. This is also not a book on writing or painting technique, acting methodology, or poetry instruction. While it is very likely that you will enjoy learning about the subject matter and will apply its insights to yourself, and that in turn will make many aspects of your life more transparent and interesting, there is no guarantee that it will.

I need to mention that in all my classes some—usually very few—students, under the impact of learning and remembering more about themselves, have needed to seek extra help. I regard this outcome as beneficial. Self-discovery is not always an easy process, and some can benefit from seeking professional help. As I discuss increasingly potent channels of access, layers of the onion will be peeled away and you may be faced with important, but sometimes difficult, self-knowledge.

One of the differences between the course and this book is that in the class, there is a sense of group cohesion among the students that will most likely not be available to you as a reader, unless of course you study this material in a group that you yourself assemble. I have had students who have continued to meet in a smaller group format, sometimes with a clinician as a leader, sometimes not, and report that they have had very interesting and helpful results. While this support can be comforting as one goes through this self-discovery journey, it is not a necessary element of the process. If however, as a reader, you find that you would benefit from in-person support, one option is to bring your psychometric test results from this book to a psychologist or psychiatrist who can provide professional guidance. It also may be helpful for professionals—psychologists, psychiatrists, in practice or in training—to create your own reading groups in order to refine your understanding of how one most successfully approaches the hidden mind. Some of our own trainees here at Stanford have found this format very helpful. However you choose to undertake this journey, I hope that you will find it rewarding, fruitful, and enlightening.

The structure of the book

I rely on both evidence-based medicine (peer reviewed papers and clinical trials) and practice-based evidence (experience with treating patients) throughout this book. Though clinical trials provide valuable information about how the human brain works, it is problematic to generalize results generated from a very specific group of people to all human beings. Trials usually focus on very minute details of the whole picture in groups of people who are assumed to be almost identical on crucial parameters (a daring assumption), and within three to four years after the publication of a scientific paper, half of its results will be proven wrong or are outdated.

I balance these limitations with insights gained from clinical practice, which focuses on the individual. This too, has its downside—the standard of evidence that emerges from treating patients is less stringent than that of clinical trials and often takes the form of "it helps," or "it works," without an attempt to control for the hundreds of variables that enter into the equation.

As a physician treating people, I must be competent and conversant in both science and clinical practice in order to blend both streams of knowledge into a tailored balance that fits the individual I am trying to help. This book attempts to show you, as a reader, how to do the same for yourself. For those of you that would like to go deeply into each topic, I will provide an overview of reading references and the most salient primary sources.

Acknowledgments

This book, like every one I have ever worked on, is of course the confluence of many people's influences, help, and concrete contributions. I would like to thank all past classes; my many patients who have given permission to use their material; my professors in psychiatry who have taught me a great deal about the centrality of psychiatry in medicine by showing me how to add psychiatric tools to the healing process (Viktor Frankl, M.D., Ph.D.; Alan Schatzberg, M.D.; Irvin Yalom, M.D.); my analytic supervisors (Saul Harrison, Thomas Szasz, Cecily Legg) who recovered from their disappointment that I did not become an analyst as they had hoped, but continued to help me understand psychodynamics and the unconscious in a deep and lasting way; the staff of the Stanford Continuing Studies Office (Alex Argyropoulos, Liz Frith, Rolando Garcia, Charles Junkerman, Dan Colman); the Winter 2012–2013 Stanford Continuing Studies PSY 199 class members; and all those who have given their feedback on this manuscript (NeuWrite; Joan Brodovsky; Rafael Pelayo, M.D.; William C. Dement, M.D., Ph.D.; Michael Greicius, M.D.; The Pegasus Physician Writers at Stanford; Kae Belgrade). All of them have helped make this book what it is. Rebecca Hall and I are very grateful.

CHAPTER ONE

Why pay attention to the unconscious? Famous artists as case studies: Rene Magritte, Artemisia Gentileschi, Georgia O'Keeffe, Egon Schiele, and Vincent van Gogh

During every moment of life, whether we are awake or asleep, our brains are orchestrating a symphony of mental, physical, and emotional processes, from our conscious thoughts of dinner plans, to the feeling of love for our children, to our rhythmic breaths. While we mostly feel in control of our thoughts, feelings, and bodies, the truth is that our brains are the true conductors of our lives, leaving us with a sense of unity as a person, but as we now know with a reasonable sense of certainty, operating completely outside of our conscious awareness 95 percent of the time. In order to comprehend and appreciate this veritable feat, we need to break down the kinds of processes we are speaking of. So it comes as no surprise that physiologic processes, such as breathing, fall into the category of unconscious mental activity. However, a vast array of emotional and cognitive activities also takes place without any conscious awareness, a fact that surprises most of us, unless of course we have studied this area of psychology or have been in a kind of therapy that takes these facts seriously. Many of these processes have significant effects on who we are and how we relate to the world. Choices, behaviors, desires, and perceptions of reality are all heavily influenced by these hidden mental activities. In effect, the unconscious mind has a great deal of influence on our conscious experience of reality.

The Unconscious:
A Modern View (John Barg. Social psychology & the unconscious:
The Automaticity of higher Mental processes. NY, Psychology press, 2007)

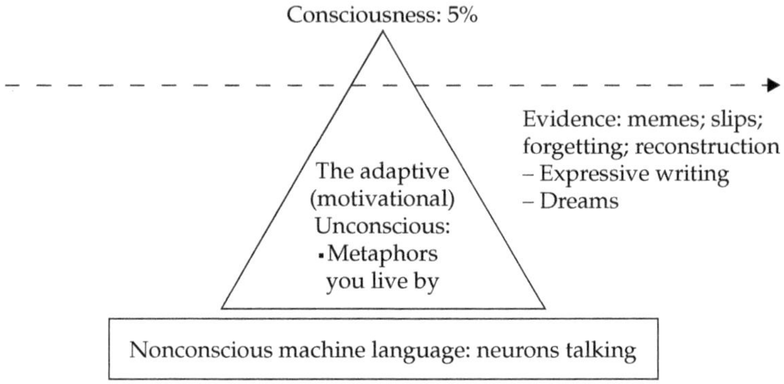

This begs the question—what secrets are our minds keeping from us? Why would this be of benefit to us? What if we could gain access to our unconscious minds and, in doing so, expand and improve our conscious experience of life? What if instead we were aware of every single little impulse, thought, belief, doubt, joy, and problematic outcome of our actions? Would we not be better for it? The obvious answer is: no. Just as we imagine the flood of information we would have to deal with in a day or even hour, we can see how having a vast reservoir of "automatic" processes that steer us according to past experiences, lessons learned, and decisions made makes for a much smoother ride through the commerce of a day. The Nobel Prize winning author, John Coetzee has recently teamed up with an English psychoanalyst to argue that it may be best to let sleeping dogs lie, if one has a reasonably good life (Coetzee & Kurtz, 2015). I would say to that: fair enough. But this is a big if. And what if sleeping dogs dream? Or even have nightmares?

Could there be circumstances when it would be good to examine what is in our unconscious? Let us pursue this thought a bit further. The unconscious serves as a reservoir of life experiences, which, even when left unexamined, significantly influences our behavior and interpretation of future experiences (Hassin, Uleman, & Bargh, 2005). For instance, someone who has faced a serious illness will consequently be likely to interpret even the most benign symptoms, such as a mild headache or a sore back, as a sign of serious illness. Because we unconsciously interpret events in light of our past experience, we often misinterpret and misperceive experiences. The result is something that in psycho-oncology we call the "Damocles syndrome": even long-term survivors of cancer are very often extremely vigilant of any aches and pains they experience. They may take them to the doctor's office far more frequently than needed, and many times such frequent complaints and worries will lead to tests and interventions which are done out of extreme caution and without any basis for real concern. Such tests can lead to all kinds of adverse outcomes. They come at a cost to the patient.

We encounter a similar scenario when we have been exposed to traumatic experiences. Veterans of war are an example often encountered, where past extreme threats to one's life leave deep scars, easily activated by the dangers of everyday living, resulting often in extreme situations in which the person or his loved ones come to harm. Such consequences are also common in survivors of accidents and family tragedies, such as premature deaths of loved ones. It therefore serves us to analyze these processes of vigilance and remedy any resulting maladaptive patterns. In doing so, we can improve our functioning, leading to happier, more fulfilling lives. If our brains are the conductors of our lives, then the more we can understand our own unconscious mental processes, the more we conduct our own symphony. After all, as Socrates so eloquently said, the unexamined life is not worth living.

One example of how the unconscious can take over and cause undesirable outcomes is from a personal experience of mine. A few years ago, my department at Stanford was interviewing professors to join the faculty. I was in charge of organizing the comings and goings of these potential new faculty members—a duty that I was happy to perform, for the most part. However, I disagreed with the university's decision to invite one individual, for I had no respect for his limited and pedestrian work. But the university would not budge, and so I put my personal feelings aside and dutifully scheduled him to give a talk here at Stanford. He happened to come on a day when we usually did not have these kinds of talks, and so I was diligent in alerting the faculty to his arrival and his scheduled presentation. In other words, I was extremely clear on the details of his presentation and diligent in making sure that my entire faculty knew and planned to be present. The day came, and as the hour of the talk approached, I remember sitting in my office making phone calls and answering emails, while the rest of the faculty attended the presentation, as I had requested. I did not consciously decide to skip the talk in protest, nor as a snub. As I made those phone calls, I was unaware of the date, the time, or where I should have been. I had absolutely no recollection of the event that I had worked so hard to organize. When the presentation had finished, the visiting professor, along with the collected faculty, walked down the hallway towards my office in order to thank me for the invitation. At that moment I remembered in full force what I had forgotten. One of our brightest faculty members, and a great friend, I might add, said with a smile, "I am sorry, Hans, that you had this emergency come up so unexpectedly," saving my face and other parts of my anatomy.

For me, this experience stands out as a prime example of how the unconscious often takes the reins. I had every conscious intention of being at that presentation despite my personal feelings towards the speaker, and yet, when the time came, my unconscious completely eliminated the entire event from my awareness. These are normative processes that happen within all of us, all the time. The question is, just how often is the unconscious at the wheel, and what happens as a result? How often does it actually play tricks on us and get us into trouble? How many times does it in fact protect us and solve problems for us? (After all, I did not have to sit through an extremely boring talk by "forgetting" its occurrence.)

In the decades since Sigmund Freud, psychologists, psychiatrists, and neuroscientists have made significant advances in understanding the complex interaction among the different layers of mentation, which can be classified into three categories: the conscious mind, the unconscious mind, and the nonconscious brain. Mental processes that exist within awareness are defined as conscious mentation. These include the thoughts, memories, desires, attitudes, beliefs, and motives that we are aware of during any particular moment. They also include the external stimuli and elements of our surroundings that we knowingly focus on. For example, if we watch a movie, our conscious processes might include the visual stimuli on the screen, the verbal dialogue, the sound of the person next to us eating popcorn, and our thoughts about the actors. Conscious processes are easily accessed, except when we are sleeping or in an altered state, such as under the influence of drugs or alcohol. As a general rule, we are able to shift our focus of attention from one aspect of conscious mentation to another, and while at times this can be effortful, access to the conscious mind is usually relatively easy.

The next layer of mental activity is the unconscious, which consists of mental processes that usually operate outside of awareness, but can be accessible and made conscious by different techniques, typically involving some form of effortful redirection of our attention and focus. Sometimes we encounter unexpected obstacles in this process (Sigmund Freud termed these as "defenses" or resistance). These are automatic processes that are very well studied in mental health. Their job is to protect us from too much anxiety and worry, or to induce in us a state of contentment and even happiness. They are very often based on the successful adaptation to past circumstances. Sometimes they solve problems for us, as we will see below, but at a minor or even major cost.

Unconscious processes are sometimes referred to as subconscious, but in this text we will adhere to the more recent terminology of unconscious. Modern neuroscience has shown us three types of unconscious processes: procedural, declarative, and motivational. The procedural unconscious refers to the memory and execution of perceptual and motor skills, like riding a bike or driving a car. For most of us, when we drive to work in the morning we don't consciously think about how to execute every action involved in driving, we just do it. This is the procedural unconscious at work.

The declarative unconscious refers to knowledge about people, places, and things. For example, the declarative unconscious remembers the facts of our lives, such as our names, families, nationality, gender, date of birth, age, and political convictions. These pieces of information are not necessarily in the forefront of our thinking, but we can readily draw upon them when we, for instance, apply for a passport.

The motivational unconscious is composed of the emotionally and experientially formed mental processes that generally exist outside of awareness but have significant effects on decisions, goals, expectations, emotional reactions, and relationships. In the above example of watching a movie, motivational unconscious processes would dictate our perceptions of the movie, how we react to it emotionally, and which elements of it we choose to focus on, such as the female or the male actors, the music in the film, or the landscape. Take for instance, the movie *Giant*. Some of us would come away with a strong impression of Elizabeth Taylor, her lack of timidity, her outspokenness, and her fearless confrontation of privilege; others would be more impressed by her incredible beauty, coyness, and passion. I leave it for you to decide which one of these impressions would be more common in young women or young men.

Impulsive, quick behaviors, like making automatic snap judgments, are particularly controlled by unconscious processes. In other words, the unconscious portion of our brain absorbs and stores information that we are not consciously aware of. Unbeknown to us, these unconscious data then manifest in how we act, think, and feel, thereby influencing a great deal of our lives. For instance, having been the victim of date rape, a young woman subsequently might attribute aggressive or even violent intent to a young man who tries to impress her by being decisive and proactive in ordering them dinner in a restaurant. This may sound ridiculous, but I have encountered many such distortions in patients in my clinical practice. Analyzing our unconscious provides insight into who we are and why we do what we do. In this book we will give the reader some tools to create a private workspace where we can develop this awareness, which then gives us the opportunity to change potentially maladaptive unconscious processes and patterns.

Very often, many manifestations of our unconscious are noticeable to others, but not necessarily to us. For example, someone else may notice that my foot is tapping frantically, suggesting I feel nervous, but I may be totally unaware of these feelings. I may even be unaware of my foot tapping. When someone points out an unconscious behavior like this, we are caught by surprise most of the time. But, as we direct our attention toward the unconscious mentation, attitude, or behavior in question, we can bring these processes into awareness. By simply shifting focus, our unconscious becomes conscious.

There are circumstances, however, in which access to the unconscious is not so easy and when gaining awareness of unconscious phenomena requires special training and tools. When aspects of the unconscious are undesirable—they may be socially inappropriate, unflattering, embarrassing, or frightening—we automatically employ defense processes that prevent us from accessing these areas of the unconscious. These defenses will be discussed in detail in Chapter Three. Defenses are one of Sigmund Freud's greatest contributions to everyday psychology. These are processes that are not lies. In fact the person being defensive is very often unaware of the fact that he is concealing things from others, because he simultaneously is concealing these very things from himself.

We all have aspects that we do not like and would rather hide from others and, indeed, from ourselves. Or we have aspects of our positive side that we would rather not acknowledge, such as our passions for other people, our enjoyment of good fortune, or our delight when a bully gets his come-uppance. We use defenses to protect ourselves from the anxiety of disapproval that these undesirable parts can cause. By relegating the negative parts of ourselves to the unconscious, we do not have to face them. However, even the areas of the unconscious that defenses prevent us from accessing leave traces in our lives, which can in turn be analyzed and provide information about us. Fortunately for us, these traces of the unconscious pop up in creative works, such as writing, painting, and acting; in psychological measures like ink blot tests and questionnaires; in expressive writing exercises; in dreams; and in relationships. These are the channels of accessing the unconscious that I will explore in this book. The reader will become familiar with these techniques in a series of exercises (Chapters Four to Seven).

The deepest layer of mental activity, nonconscious mentation, is comprised of neuronal processes and activities that are probably never accessible to awareness, regardless of the length of introspection, meditation, or mindfulness. These processes are deeply embedded in the billions of neurons in the brain, and no matter how much effort we exert or how much psychological analysis we undertake, the majority of nonconscious mentation can never be made conscious. We can, however, get glimpses of these processes using scientific instrumentation, such as electroencephalography (the recording of electrical activity in the brain) and functional imaging, and with psychophysiological measures, such as lie detector tests and biofeedback machines.

Sometimes, these nonconscious processes control external manifestations, such as heart rate. Certain people can learn to consciously regulate some of these nonconscious processes through extensive focused attention and specialized training methods, like meditation and yoga. However, even those most experienced in these techniques can only control nonconscious processes within fairly firm limits, which are usually given by Mother Nature, our genetic endowment, and epigenetic development. While some may be able to use meditation to slow down their racing heart, no one will be able to consciously stop his heart from beating, regardless of how much he concentrates. In reality, the boundary between unconscious and nonconscious processes is more fluid than the line I have drawn here and will likely change as our understanding of the mind and brain improves. There is already some evidence that specialized techniques can alter this boundary. Yoga and meditation are good examples of how learned skills can be used to control nonconscious processes in ways that we are usually incapable of. However, in this discussion I address only those skills used to access the unconscious mind and therefore maintain a distinction between unconscious and nonconscious processes. These techniques that aim to control the nonconscious mind lie outside of the scope of this text and will not be discussed or taught here. I will limit this discussion to the handling of unconscious material.

Some prefer to leave the mystery of the unconscious alone rather than explore what may be lurking beneath the surface (see my comments above regarding the 2015 book *The Good Story* by Coetzee and Kurtz). We now will turn to a great example that shows concretely that sleeping dogs may not remain eternally dormant, no matter how much we may want them to do so. The artwork of Rene Magritte illustrates how the motivational unconscious manifests in our actions, whether we like it or not. To be clear, we are not making the claim here that Magritte was such an accomplished artist because of his unconscious; his talent would have been present regardless of his experiences. However, some of his experiences left traces in the content of his art, which told and at the same time disguised the traumatic events that could not fail to impact a developing youngster. His virtuosity probably helped him to keep the impact of his traumatic past under some control. But as his regretful remark at the end of his life indicates, keeping the demons dormant incurred a cost.

The unconscious at work—Rene Magritte

A quick preamble to this portion of the book: In class we spend a great deal of time letting the paintings of the artists we discuss have their effect on us. We hope the reader will find time to do the same. Almost all the paintings discussed in this section are readily available in one form or another in books, museums, and of course on the internet. Simply entering the titles of the paintings and the last name of the painter into a search engine in our experience very quickly will bring up the images we discuss. We thought of giving specific links to the pictures, but given the fluidity of the net this seems not useful. We therefore decided on the process followed from here on. As far as the pieces of art in the remainder of the book are concerned, these are all images for which we have received informed consent to reproduce.

Rene Magritte was a famous Belgian surrealist painter (November 21, 1898–August 15, 1967). He is known for images that challenge our sense of reality through unusual juxtapositions and scenes of the ordinary placed in unexpected contexts. The sometimes exacting realism of his images underlines and highlights the impossibility of the circumstances he depicted, a common surrealist agenda. In this sense, Magritte was very much a man of his time and a man of the surrealist movement. However, when looked at closely, many of Magritte's paintings also contain a deeper layer of meaning that begins to reveal the inner workings of his unconscious mind.

To examine this, I use hermeneutics, which is a way of interpreting human behavior, thoughts, and creative works, much like the way the themes and metaphors in a book or poem are read and interpreted. Looking at his paintings, we must go beyond the obvious elements of the image and interpret what significance the symbols may hold. We pay attention to the emotional undercurrent of each piece and investigate what themes, symbols, and emotionality repeat and emerge as a trend throughout his artistic career. Early on, Magritte painted predominately female nudes, many of which were of his wife, Georgette Berger. These works are slightly abstract, such as *Nude* (1919), and are classical artistic celebrations of the female body.

While evocative, there is little mystery in these works. Then, in the 1920s, he entered a new surrealist creative direction and began to paint pieces that are quite different from his early works, both in imagery and emotionality. As we continue the hermeneutic process of analysis, we see Magritte's unconscious creeping into his works, giving us insight into what may have been lurking beneath his conscious awareness.

In *The Difficult Crossing* (1926), we see a bedpost standing in the middle of a room. Next to it is a table with a severed hand holding a red dove. Planks of wood with squares cut out are strewn about the room, a brown piece of fabric hangs from the ceiling, and through the window are a dark and stormy ocean, a black sky, and fierce lightning. The overall tone of the piece is dark, tumultuous, and unnerving.

The stormy background and bedposts are repeated in *The Face of Genius* (1926), with the added element of a white, lifeless head in between the bedposts. Pieces of the face are cut out, and the one remaining eye is closed. Again, the tone is dark and threatening.

In *Le Supplice de la Vestale* (1926), a new symbol appears—a white piece of fabric draped around the shoulders of a headless, nude female torso. White spikes protrude from the top of the torso's neck, and, again, an ominous ocean lurks in the background.

The white fabric shows up again in *The Dawn of Cayenne* (1926), which depicts a pair of severed hands wrapped in the fabric and holding an eerie red spider. Next to the hands is a single candle, and in the background are barren branches. The images in this piece all suggest lifelessness—the severed hands, the bare branches, and the candle, an item typically found at funerals.

When contemplating these pieces, do you feel comforted, calm, and joyful, or are you disquieted? For many of us, these images are disturbing. They are filled with torment, and the interplay between the comfort of pedestrian realism and the turmoil of unexpected juxtapositions elicits feelings of threat, unease, and fear. Having identified a repeating emotional tone and constellation of symbols, we begin to wonder about the source of these emotions within Magritte and what meaning the imagery may hold.

Moving forward in Magritte's repertoire, we come to *The Musings of a Solitary Walker* (1926). What appears to be a female, nude corpse lies in the foreground, and a man wearing Magritte's characteristic black jacket and bowler hat stands with his back to her. To the left is a river with a bridge, set underneath a threatening sky.

These themes persist with even more explicit imagery in his works throughout 1927. Rarely, though, are these paintings portrayed in a completely straightforward manner. If explicit, they usually contain a large element of surrealism, which in turn disguises and negates the outright, straightforward depiction of violent events.

The Menaced Assassin (1927) is a good example of this style. Here, a disturbing murder scene is depicted in a highly surrealistic manner. In the foreground are two threatening men lurking just outside a room, one with a net, and the other with a club. In the room, a naked woman lies dead on a bed, her head severed. She has blood dripping from her mouth and a white cloth draped over her neck. A man stands in the room with his back to the body, somewhat relaxed and listening to a phonograph. Three other men stare into the room from a window in the background.

The facts of the scene are unquestionably violent—a corpse, a severed head, and captors lurking in the shadows, waiting to attack the presumed assassin. However, these violent images are directly contrasted with elements of calm and peace. Snow capped mountain peaks are visible through the window in the background. A few feet away from the corpse, the man calmly listens to music with his coat and hat nonchalantly draped over a chair, as one might do when alone in a quiet room. The effect of this juxtaposition is a minimization of the violent and disturbing elements of the scene, though the painting still elicits an ominous and unsettling feeling. What seems calm is not, or is it? Would you want to enter this room?

In 1928, the draped white fabric that we previously saw in *Le Supplice de la Vestale* and *The Dawn of Cayenne* reappears in a number of pieces. In *The Lovers*, two white sheets cover the heads of a man and a woman. In *The Symmetrical Trick*, a white sheet hangs over the torso of a female nude, leaving the lower half of her body exposed. White sheets hang on either side, giving the appearance of concealed heads. In *The Heart of the Matter* the same cloth is draped over a human head; in *The Invention of Life* it covers an entire figure—an image reminiscent of a ghost. The repeated use of the white cloth suggests that it is a particularly meaningful symbol for Magritte. The question is, why?

In *Attempting the Impossible* (1928) we see Magritte painting a female figure, as if he were bringing her to life. Again, she is nude. The viewer is left wondering, who is it that Magritte is trying to recreate?

Later in his career, he begins to hint at the answer to this question. In *The Spirit of Geometry* (1937), an adult figure holds a baby. However, the heads have been switched—the adult body has a child's head, and the baby has been painted with the mother's head—suggesting a role reversal and calling into question who is taking care of whom. The baby is draped in the recurring white cloth.

In his 1940 painting *Homesickness*, a man with black wings leans against the side of a bridge, looking out and over the edge. Behind him sits a lion. The lion and the man have their backs to each other, each gazing out in opposite directions. The man's all black attire in combination with his black wings is reminiscent of the angel of death, while the presence of a lion adds an ominous, but powerful, feeling. A yellow haze in the air makes it difficult to time the event. The scene has an inferred timelessness, a feeling that sometimes comes to us at moments of great shock. As a whole, it evokes a feeling of melancholy. The title of the painting, *Homesickness*, corroborates the general mood of sadness created by the image.

The scene is set on a bridge, presumably over a river—another recurring theme. When the same images continue to appear in multiple works, they are likely to be personally significant. There is a reason that Magritte chooses to focus on rivers, consciously or unconsciously.

These themes of death and violence persist in many of his paintings as time progresses. In 1947, he painted *Philosophy in the Boudoir*, in which a white nightgown with nude breasts hangs in a closet. This makes the garment look like a ghost-like, headless body.

In 1948 he produced *Memory*, which shows a lifeless, battered female head with blood above her right eye. The background is another body of water.

Later in his career, Magritte produced pieces that still sometimes evoke dark and threatening emotionality, but predominately call into question our sense of reality. In *The Empire of Light* (1950) he accomplishes this by juxtaposing images of night and day. In this painting, a blue sky full of bright clouds is set against the darkness of night in the street below. Underneath a daytime sky, the building windows glow from within, and a single streetlamp shines into the darkness. The concurrence of night and day leaves us disoriented and disquieted. Would you enter one of these houses, or would you be hesitant to do so? A theme of threat and danger is paradoxically transmitted in beautiful form.

He continued to challenge what is real and what is not with *This Is Not an Apple* (1964), which depicts an apple together with the inscription, "This is not an apple." At first look, the title seems contradictory—the painting clearly shows an apple. However, upon further analysis the statement is actually correct. The painting is not a real, physical apple; we cannot reach out and take a bite out of it. The painting is an *image* of an apple. Here, Magritte brings into question the relationship between words, images, and objects, ultimately challenging the convention of identifying an image as the object itself—what is real, and what is actually only our comprehension of reality? Where is the line between reality, fantasy, and fiction? And why was Magritte so preoccupied with playing with the boundary between reality and fantasy?

Magritte's personal history offers a window of insight into the motivation behind these paintings and answers many of the questions that his works have raised. Throughout Magritte's childhood, his mother, Regina Bertinchamp, suffered from depression, and she attempted suicide several times. Then, in 1912, she disappeared in the middle of the night. She shared a bed with her youngest child, Paul, who had awakened and realized that she was gone. The family searched in vain until they noticed footprints leading to the bridge over the Sambre River. Bertinchamp had jumped off the bridge in her nightgown and drowned. Fourteen-year-old Magritte later watched as his mother's body was fished out of the river with her wet, tangled nightgown—the white cloth—pulled up and over her face. Her naked body was badly bruised and battered.

In *Homesickness*, the angel of death figure standing on the edge of a bridge now holds particular significance given the nature of his mother's suicide. *The Spirit of Geometry* also begins to make sense in this context—children of depressed parents often experience feelings of role reversal, believing that they must be the ones to take care of the adult. Likewise, the violent scene in *The Menaced Assassin* takes on a new understanding. The nude female corpse with a white cloth draped over her neck could be a representation of Magritte's mother. Troubled waters, bridges, bedposts, and the nightgown appear over and over again, often in conjunction with veiled faces, female nudes, and symbols of death.

The pieces that question our perception of reality also take on a new meaning given the context of her death. A young child who witnesses the sudden death of his mother would be expected to struggle to make sense of the event. Having his concept of life and family shattered at such a young age would likely lead to a preoccupation with questioning reality.

The images in these works are not only symbolic of the events surrounding Bertinchamp's suicide, the paintings also evoke dark and unsettling emotions in us as viewers—emotions that we may have expected Magritte to experience as a result of the tragedy. These are a small sample of such paintings; Magritte's pieces are filled with symbols, imagery, and emotionality that correlate to his mother's death.

It is no coincidence that, as a young boy, Magritte witnessed the tragic death of his mother and, as an adult, he continually placed violent themes and unsettling images in his paintings. Magritte, however, protested the correlation between the symbolism in his paintings and his traumatic childhood. He himself described his paintings as "visible images which conceal nothing; they evoke mystery and, indeed, when one sees one of my pictures, one asks oneself this simple question, 'What does that mean?' It does not mean anything, because mystery means nothing either, it is unknowable." When asked what lay "behind" one of his paintings, he responded, "There is nothing 'behind' this image.

Behind the paint of the painting there is the canvas. Behind the canvas there is a wall. Behind the wall there is … etc. Visible things always hide other visible things. But a visible image hides nothing." The images that he painted are heavily laden with symbolism that indicates memories of his childhood emotional trauma, and yet he did not believe that the content of his paintings carried any particular significance.

Magritte resisted the analysis of his artwork to such a degree that we can even see this attitude creep into some of his paintings. In 1951 he produced *Perspective: Madame Récamier by David,* which shows a coffin reclining in a chair. The white sheet appears again here, tucked underneath the coffin. We can interpret this piece as another memory of his mother's death, but the image is also reminiscent of a psychotherapy session in which the patient typically lies on a couch. When viewed in this light, it can be seen as an affront to the idea of analyzing his paintings for underlying meaning. As one of my students so aptly said, the piece seems to be saying, "You can psychoanalyze me over my dead body." This attitude was persistent throughout Magritte's life. Sigmund Freud supposedly offered to analyze him for free—an offer which he roundly rejected. And as late as 1948, in an interview with André Gomez for Radio Suisse Romande, we can see him fending off any and all questions by the interviewer to categorize him in any way, and insisting on the unconscious, automatic nature of his art: "Ah well, don't you see that I had no choice (in deciding to paint), no more than I could chose the color of my hair. It happened. I don't know how it happened. I have always painted. I really don't remember how it came about." Magritte's refusal to engage in any form of discourse with the interviewer that even approaches narrative and meaning is pervasive throughout the interview, regardless of what question is asked. It is as if he said: above all, attribute no meaning to anything I (and others) do. The world goes on with or without any of us understanding what is happening. This attitude seems quite puzzling to all of us that constantly ask ourselves questions about our purpose, the meaning of life, etc. It only can be understood if one comprehends its larger purpose in Magritte's life, which was to protect him from sadness, anxiety, or perhaps even guilt in relationship to his mother's suicide.

Magritte's inability to see the influence of his mother's death on his work is likely related to his reluctance to admit the impact the tragedy had on his own psyche. Many years later, during a conversation with his close friend, Louis Scutenaire, Magritte claimed that the only feeling he remembers in connection with his mother's suicide is "one of intense pride at the thought of being the pitiable center of attention in a drama." Imagine, for a moment, that at the young age of fourteen you discover your mother's body washed up on a shore. Would the singular emotion produced by this experience be one of pride? Would you be excited about being a part of the drama, devoid of all other emotion surrounding your mother's tragic death? Most of us would expect a young adolescent faced with this situation to be overcome with a range of complex emotions, such as grief and anger. Magritte, on the other hand, remembers feeling only pride. And yet, his artwork is rife with the emotion we would expect after a trauma. Magritte may have resisted feeling or acknowledging these emotions consciously, but that did not mean that they did not exist within him.

Magritte's paintings exemplify how the unconscious mind manifests in our actions and, more specifically, in our artistic expressions. T. S. Eliot coined a term for such a relationship—objective correlative—in his essay "Hamlet and His Problems." While Magritte remained consciously unaware of the effect that his mother's death had on him, his artwork suggests significant emotional trauma. Because he resisted experiencing the emotions surrounding the event, they lay hidden, but not dormant, in his motivational unconscious and eventually bubbled up to the surface in the form of his artwork. While it may not have been his conscious, deliberate intention to paint about the death of his mother, his unconscious mental processes motivated him to do so. I will discuss the use of art as a vehicle to enter the unconscious further in Chapter Five.

Later in life, Magritte noted that he regretted his preoccupation with images of violence and trauma. In 1946 he signed a manifesto, *Surrealism in Full Sunlight*, which renounced the violence and pessimism in his earlier work and proposed "a search for joy and pleasure." As accomplished and admired as Magritte was, in his eyes he had significant limits to his creativity. As he said himself, "Between ourselves, it is terrible what one lays oneself open to when drawing an innocent picture." This was the price he paid for using his artistic gift to control and sublimate his experience, instead of allowing his experience to fully integrate into his consciousness, let grief run its course, and achieve more conscious closure on the way his mother died. It is quite obvious that Magritte was an exceptional artist despite his preoccupations. It is also clear that his talent existed outside of his traumatic experiences.

In other words, his trauma did not cause his creative talent. But his trauma narrowed the content of what he was to achieve. Who knows what he might have accomplished, had he not found it necessary to dedicate one third of his *oeuvre* to keeping the demons at bay. Again, in his interview with Gomez in 1948, he said, "Listen, I think I probably wouldn't have painted in the style I use now, but I think I would still have tried to create new sensations."

Artemisia Gentileschi

The main unconscious theme in Magritte's work had to do with his reaction to and the recapitulation of his imaginings regarding his mother's tragic death. In Artemisia's work, we will encounter a different theme—one equally stirring and disturbing, but of a different emotional quality.

Artemisia Gentileschi (1593–1656) was a celebrated Italian Baroque painter known for her dramatic artwork that often focused on women, sexuality, and violence. For example, in 1610, Artemisia painted *Susanna and the Elders* based on the Book of Daniel in the Bible. In the story, two elders secretly watch Susanna bathe and then threaten to falsely accuse her of meeting a young man unless she sleeps with them. Refusing to be blackmailed, Susanna is arrested and almost put to death before Daniel saves her. Artemisia's 1610 painting shows a nude Susanna sitting on concrete steps while the two older men hover over her. One man is whispering in the other's ear, while the second man talks to Susanna—presumably threatening her. Susanna's head is turned down and away from the men, and she has an expression of anguish on her face. Her hands are up and look as if she is trying to protect herself from the two men. The two men are conspiring. Susanna is being betrayed and threatened, but she is not taking action on her behalf.

Then, Artemisia painted *Judith Slaying Holofernes* (1611–1612). In the Book of Judith in the Bible, Judith uses her beauty to gain entry into the tent of a general named Holofernes, who was going to destroy Judith's home city. Holofernes let it be known that he would spare the city if Judith would share his bed with him. Instead, Judith decapitates Holofernes after he gets drunk and passes out. She then carries his head away in a basket. Artemisia's depiction of this story is graphic and detailed, showing Judith cutting off Holofernes' head with the help of another woman. Holofernes' blood spills onto the white sheets of a bed; Judith's expression is merciless. This story repeatedly emerges in Artemisia's artwork, with multiple renditions of the beheading scene. In other paintings, the two women are carrying Holofernes' head away in the basket (*Judith and Her Maidservant*, 1612–1613) or cleaning up the scene of the crime by candlelight (*Judith and Her Maidservant*, 1625–1628). This scene had been the theme of many paintings by male painters before Artemisia, but she added a graphic detail to the scene hitherto unknown. And she showed Judith triumphant, not repentant or frightened. Judith is someone who knows how to take care of herself and her city.

In *Mary Magdalene* (1616–1617), Artemisia shows Mary Magdalene, a prominent figure in Christianity, sitting in a bright yellow dress with the fabric sliding down one shoulder. Her right hand is clutching her heart, and she has a pained expression on her face. Mary Magdalene was depicted by the Church as a repentant prostitute during the Middle Ages. Mary Magdalene is not proud of her sexuality.

Artemisia painted *Lucretia* in 1621, which depicts the legendary Roman matron who was raped by an Etruscan king's son and consequently committed suicide. In Artemisia's rendition, Lucretia is sitting with a knife in her hand. Her face is turned up, and her right hand holds her left breast. There is a feeling of torment in the piece. Yet another victimized woman, who reacts to the wrong done to her with an extreme act of defiance. Rather than suffering the shame of her victimization, she will sacrifice herself and move beyond the bounds of traditional society.

In *David and Bathsheba* (1636–1638), Artemisia shows Bathsheba bathing in a courtyard. She has a piece of white cloth draped over her lap. One woman combs her long, wavy hair, while another offers her jewelry. A third kneels at her feet with a basin of water. In the Hebrew Bible, King David lusts after Bathsheba after seeing her bathe. He summons her to him and impregnates her. Bathsheba, however, is already married to Uriah the Hittite. To cover up their sin, King David sends Uriah to the front lines of battle, where he dies. King David then marries Bathsheba. This is yet another story of a woman not in control of her sexuality, her body, or her fate.

These are just a few examples of similar themes that dominate Artemisia's artwork. Over 50 percent of her paintings are of Susanna, Judith, Bathsheba, Lucretia, or Mary Magdalene, which are all stories that focus on themes like betrayal, rape, murder, violence, revenge, lust, or sexuality. About ten percent of her paintings are specifically of beheadings. While Artemisia was not the only artist to create artwork based on these stories and women, her depictions were particularly vivid. She also produced paintings that centered on more pleasant themes, but she was clearly preoccupied with violence, sexuality, and enraged women getting revenge on men. Why?

Artemisia was the oldest child of the Tuscan painter, Orazio Gentileschi. Her mother had died in 1605. Artemisia was a gifted painter, and in 1611, Orazio hired another painter, Agostino Tassi, to privately tutor Artemisia. Tassi then raped Artemisia. Following the rape, Artemisia continued to be intimate with Tassi under the assumption that they would marry. Tassi, however, heard a rumor that she was sleeping with another man and used this rumor to break his promise to her—a second major betrayal.

When Tassi refused to marry Artemisia, her father, Orazio, pressed charges. The trial against Tassi lasted for seven months. Artemisia, quite in contrast to many women at the time and even now, agreed to be part of that trial, knowing that what awaited her was anything but pleasant, and potentially life threatening. She was not a shrinking violet. Tassi had already faced charges for incest with his sister-in-law and had also intended to steal paintings from Orazio. Still, Tassi denied the rape accusations, and in turn claimed that Artemisia had a long history of having multiple lovers—including her father. Artemisia maintained that she had never slept with any man except for Tassi. In order to determine when she had lost her virginity, Artemisia was given a gynecological exam as part of the trial. She was also tortured with thumbscrews. To see if she was lying or telling the truth, she was further tortured with ropes that were tied tightly around her hands. As they pulled the ropes and asked her over and over if Tassi had raped her, she responded that he had. Tassi was sentenced, but escaped punishment.

It is easy to imagine the anger that Artemisia probably felt, first at being raped, then at having the promise of marriage broken, then at having to endure the public shame and physical torture of the trial, and finally at her father for failing to protect her all along. It was he who had arranged for her to be tutored by a man with a checkered past. Artemisia's artwork suggests that she may indeed have already felt betrayed by her father even before the incident with Tassi—she painted *Susanna and the Elders* (1610), which shows a young woman trying to protect herself from two older men, before the rape and trial. Perhaps she knew that her father was allowing a man with a bad reputation into their home, and she felt exposed to harm. Paintings like *Judith Slaying Holofernes*, which she created during and after the trial, confirm her anger and reveal a thirst for revenge.

Because Artemisia was repeatedly betrayed by the men in her life and sexually violated, she largely focused on painting images of women. She depicted some of these women distraught and in pain; others were powerful figures who stood up to men. Incidentally, the name Artemisia comes from "Artemis"—the Greek God of Hunting. In general, Artemisia's artwork suggests that she unconsciously harbored a desire to hunt men, a desire which she could express through her craft. Her paintings consequently oozed with rage against men.

For more information about Artemisia, there are several publications that have been produced about her (Cohen, 2000; Greer, 1979) and movies (*Artemisia*, 1997; *Artemisia: Una Donna Appassionata*, 2012), which essentially expand on the themes outlined here.

Georgia O'Keeffe

Lest we give the reader the impression that only extremely negative events and emotions get stored in our unconscious and influence our creativity for many years, let us turn to some more positive and happier traces in a painter's *oeuvre*. Georgia O'Keeffe (November 15, 1887–March 6, 1986) was an American painter known for her landscapes and large-scale depictions of flowers. She was born in Sun Prairie, Wisconsin as the second of seven children. She attended the Art Institute of Chicago in 1905 and the Art Students League in New York in 1907. In 1908 her talent began to gain recognition, and she won the Art Students League Chase scholarship for her still life painting, *Rabbit and Copper Pot* (1907).

In 1912 she was significantly influenced by Arthur Wesley Dow's idea that the goal of creating art is to express the artist's emotions and ideas. This is similar to T. S. Eliot's objective correlative. She was so struck by this idea that she destroyed most of her early work. She then started drawing a series of abstract charcoals in 1915, like *No. 12 Special* (1916). These are some of the most recognized pieces of American art from that time period.

In 1916 her life took another important turn when she began corresponding with Alfred Stieglitz, a famous photographer. She moved to New York in 1918, where she painted for a year with his funding and posed as a model for his photography. They were married in 1924. Stieglitz recognized her talent and became one of her greatest supporters throughout her career, promoting and exhibiting her artwork. In 1929, she began spending her summers painting in New Mexico, where she found a new palate that influenced her artwork. Stieglitz died in 1946, and three years later she moved from New York to New Mexico. O'Keeffe retired in 1984 due to failing eyesight.

By the mid 1920s, O'Keeffe had developed her signature style: large, close-up flowers and landscapes that are filled with feminine imagery. In *Lake George* (1922), for example, a blue mountain ridgeline is reflected in a lake. At first glance, the mountains are the subject matter of the painting. On closer inspection, the viewer sees that the outline of the mountains closely resembles the silhouette of a nude woman lying down, with the peaks and valleys tracing her curves. O'Keeffe also painted a number of magnified flowers, like *Music Pink and Blue II* (1918), *Grey Lines with Black, Blue and Yellow* (1923), *Red Canna* (1924), and *Flower of Life II* (1925). These paintings are brightly colored, close-up, detailed studies of flowers—and are highly symbolic of the female body.

Stieglitz recognized the sexual undertones of her paintings—and he understood that this brought potential buyers into the gallery. O'Keeffe resisted this idea. Her intent was not to paint provocative and scandalous paintings. She claimed that her paintings only reflected the world exactly as she saw it. In 1926, she said, "… one rarely takes the time to really see a flower. I have painted what each flower is to me and I have painted it big enough so that others would see what I see." In psychology, this type of reasoning would be called rationalization—a defense that, like many others, keeps threatening mental content from awareness and closes it off from further discussion or exploration.

If she didn't consciously intend to hide the female body in her landscapes and flowers, why did she? O'Keeffe began painting at a time when men were considered superior to women, and the artwork of female painters was not frequently exhibited. Even when praising her work, male critics made comments like "Here are masculine qualities in great variety and reserve" (Alan Burroughs, *The New York Sun*, 1923). In effect, they were saying that she was only good because she was painting like a man. O'Keeffe was determined to show the world that women were every bit as capable and talented as men. She wanted to be taken seriously as a woman in the arts, and she wanted to achieve success on her own terms. One can see her fierce determination in a 1923 portrait of O'Keeffe by Stieglitz, which shows her squarely facing the camera, eyes narrowed, jaw set, chin slightly turned up, as if to say, "Bring it on, men."

In some ways, O'Keeffe was a woman of her generation, but the motivation behind her artwork goes deeper than that. Remember the objective correlative that so deeply resonated with her—the idea that art should reflect the artist's ideas? Because she wanted to prove that women could be world-class painters, she unconsciously saw the live-giving power of femininity in all of her subject matter, and this came through in her paintings. Even as she consciously intended to create a flower or a mountain, her unconscious mind infused a heavy dose of feminine strength, sensuality, and even sexuality, into the images. Her drive to prove herself unconsciously seeped into the style of her art as she created landscapes and flowers that celebrated the power, fertility, and beauty of women.

O'Keeffe is an example of how the unconscious mind can influence artwork in a positive way. Her story is not one of trauma, betrayal, or mental illness, but rather it is one of strength. She refused to be held back by limiting societal views on gender, and this statement significantly—albeit unconsciously—influenced her artwork. By emphasizing the female form and its reflection in nature in a large majority of her works, she told the world that she could go head to head with any male artist. Still, her pride and interest in her sensual-sexual self managed to seep through to her paintings, as many critics and above all her supporter, Stieglitz, accurately identified. She rejected the idea that one should exploit these characteristics in order to keep her competitive edge in a world dominated by men.

Egon Schiele

Egon Schiele (June 12, 1890–October 31, 1918) is another example of how one's life experiences seep into artistic creations. Schiele was an Austrian figurative painter known for intense and often highly sexual portraits, many with twisted and emaciated body shapes. Going through the hermeneutic process of analysis again, let's take a look at a few of his pieces and see if we can identify any recurring themes or emotional undertones that could help us understand Schiele's unconscious.

Take his 1910 self-portrait, for example. Is this painting warm and inviting, or does it put you on guard? Schiele's angular posture, arms, and fingers combined with the harsh brush strokes, sickly colors, and menacing facial expression create a threatening tone. This portrait does not look like a healthy, happy person.

In another self-portrait from 1911, Schiele angles his head and turns up his nose. He looks like he is analyzing and judging his world, as though everything is beneath him. His raised eyebrows and widened eyes create a feeling of questioning or doubt. His skeleton-like fingers are posed in a V—odd hand gestures are a recurring symbol in many of his works—though we aren't sure why, or what it means. The V seems like a secret code that we are not privy to. We get the feeling that Schiele is saying, "I know something you don't know, and I'm not going to tell you." There is a distinct feeling of distance between Schiele and the viewer in this painting, as if he is superior. He looks disdainful, and the tone is cold.

The Self Seers II (Death and Man) (1911) exemplifies another pervasive theme throughout Schiele's paintings—death. In this frightening picture, a figure wearing all black stands in the foreground. Its face looks stripped of skin, and its expression is menacing and haunting. A fearful figure dressed in white stands behind him. Again, we see the skeleton-like hands.

A large portion of Schiele's artistic repertoire consists of paintings and drawings of nude or partially nude females. In *Lying, Half-Dressed Girl* (1911), for example, we see a woman lying down with her eyes closed, naked from the waist up. Much like the 1910 self-portrait shown above, she does not look healthy and full of life. She looks fragile, even ill, and her expression feels sad.

Many of Schiele's female nudes depict women in suggestive or outright pornographic poses, like *Kneeling Woman with Head Bent Forward* (1915), which shows a woman bending forward at the waist with disheveled clothing. She hides her face, perhaps out of shame or fear. The painting feels chaotic.

Schiele's focus on sexuality and nudity continues in paintings like *Act of Love* (1915). Here we see a man and a woman in an intimate pose. The man is on top of the woman and seems to engulf her with his body; the picture feels claustrophobic. Again, the subjects do not look healthy. The colors are insipid, sickly, and there appear to be bruises on the skin of both man and woman. Neither is looking at the other—there is no eye contact—instead each stares to the side with a lifeless expression. This is not a happy or exciting depiction of intimacy.

Schiele's paintings were considered particularly shocking and pornographic in the early twentieth century, and some continue to find his pieces disturbing. Why was Schiele so focused on producing provocative and controversial art filled with sex, death, and doubt?

When Schiele was a boy, his father, Adolf Schiele, was the stationmaster of the Tulln station in the Austrian State Railways, a respectable position in society. But when Schiele was fifteen years old, his father's honorable façade was shattered when he died from syphilis, a disease commonly contracted from prostitutes during that time period. Due to his societal status, his father's illness and its cause would likely have been unacknowledged until almost the very end of his life, even though symptoms like dementia had emerged—he burned the family fortune because he wanted to make a fire, for example. Not long after his father's death, Schiele began studying art.

His father's illness and death unveiled the discrepancy between his honorable standing within the community and his dishonorable secret behavior. On the one hand Schiele's father was an upright, respected citizen, but behind closed doors he was a man that paid women for sex. Such dual lives were pervasive in Vienna during that time. The Austrian aristocracy coexisted with a strong, unspoken culture of women selling themselves. Many were growing dissatisfied with the Austrian monarchy and the hypocrisy of its culture. Schiele's artwork suggests that he, likewise, developed a mistrustful, disdainful view of the world.

As an artist trying to build a career, Schiele could not be openly critical of the aristocracy. But he could use his paintings as an outlet for his dissent. By painting women in lewd poses, he challenged the secret immorality of the publicly respected gentry. His judgmental attitude toward society also shows up in his self-portraits, which repeatedly show him with a scornful, superior facial expression and posture. He looks doubtful—perhaps that the formality and apparent morality that surround him are real. The secret code that we noted in the position of his hands could reflect this perspective—he knows the unspoken truth of the world: people are not what they pretend to be.

Schiele's experiences also show up in his artwork in subtle ways that may have been unconscious. He tended to paint figures that look sickly—a possible reflection of his father's illness and death. Schiele realized that life is difficult and full of threats, and his art consequently contains a pervasive sadness. *The Self Seers II (Death and Man)* (1911) takes on a new meaning given his father's illness. The two figures, one in white and one black, mirror the two sides of a double life: the honorable and the dishonorable, the man with morals and the man who visits prostitutes. His preoccupation with nude females and sad or threatening depictions of intimacy may also reflect the nature of his father's illness. Rather than a caring act of love, intimacy was a secret, shameful act that hurt Schiele's father, and ultimately killed him.

Schiele may not have experienced a traumatic childhood event like Magritte did—the nature of the death of Schiele's father was not so unusual during that time period—but his life experience still colored his artwork, perhaps in ways that even Schiele, himself, did not realize. Much like Magritte's trauma narrowed the focus of his art to symbols that related to his mother's death, Schiele's experiences constricted the focus of his art to predominately illness, sex, and death.

Vincent van Gogh

Vincent van Gogh (March 30, 1853–July 29, 1890) was a Postimpressionist painter who is now one of the most famous artists in the world. Most people are familiar with his iconic artwork, like *Starry Night* (1889), and his tragic personal life—he cut off his ear and ended his own life. It is widely accepted that he suffered from a mental illness, though there is ongoing debate about his particular diagnosis. Rather than arguing the specifics of his psychiatric condition here, I include Van Gogh in the present discussion as a final example of how one's life experiences and emotions can filter into artwork. Let's go through the hermeneutic process of analysis one more time with a few of his paintings to see how his story emerges from the canvas.

In 1887, while living in Paris, Van Gogh painted *Self-Portrait with Grey Felt Hat*. In it, we see Van Gogh with his characteristic red beard wearing a grey hat, dark blue jacket, and staring straight into the viewer's eyes. What are you reminded of when you look at the prominent yellow and orange stripes on Van Gogh's face, painted in a concentric circle out from his nose? The brush strokes look like a tiger's stripes or war paint, giving Van Gogh a fierce appearance. His eyes are stern, almost angry, with a hint of sadness. The deep blue hues contribute to the painting's serious tone.

This self-portrait gives a clear sense of his anger at the lack of recognition he received for his talents. Van Gogh was a starving artist. He was poor, lived off of financial support from his younger brother, Theo, and he struggled to sell paintings even though Theo was an art dealer. Of the more than 2000 artworks that he created, he only sold one painting during his lifetime. When he made *Self-Portrait with Grey Felt Hat*, he had not sold a single piece. We can feel his frustration in the painting.

In February of 1888, he moved to Arles to escape Paris, feeling worn down and ill from excessive alcohol consumption and smoking. Some say he moved to Arles with the hope of founding a utopian art colony. In October of 1888, he painted *Bedroom in Arles*, which shows his small, but orderly, bedroom. Everything is in its place; it does not feel chaotic. There are no strong emotional undertones. Perhaps Van Gogh was beginning to feel more settled when he painted this. He may have been looking forward to the prospect of starting an art colony with his friends. But take a closer look at the painting: its perspective is slightly off—the room feels shaky and unstable, as if the floor might waver at any minute and tip the furniture over. Van Gogh was still not on solid ground.

Paul Gauguin, another Postimpressionist painter whom Van Gogh and Theo had befriended in Paris, visited Van Gogh in Arles. Van Gogh admired Gauguin and hoped that he would stay in Arles to help build the art colony, but things did not go as Van Gogh planned. Their relationship deteriorated, and tensions rose as Van Gogh realized that Gauguin planned to leave Arles. Though the details of the situation remain debated, one night in December of 1888, the two had an argument, and Van Gogh sliced off his ear lobe with a razor. He then bandaged his wound, wrapped the severed ear in paper, and left it at a brothel for safekeeping. He returned home and collapsed. The next day he was found unconscious and taken to the hospital. He recovered but continued to suffer from delusions, and two months later he left Arles to enter an asylum.

While in the clinic, he painted *The Starry Night* (June of 1889). In this famous painting, a town sits beneath a swirling night sky, creating a feeling of movement. A bright, crescent moon is in the upper right hand corner, the sky is filled with large, yellow stars, and a black cypress tree dominates the foreground on the left hand side. The contours of the cypress tree mirror the whirling night. The town feels sleepy and quiet, a juxtaposition that makes the night sky feel even more dramatic.

The sky is turbulent and troubled; this is not a calm scene. Darkness is descending.

Van Gogh stayed in the asylum for a year. In September of 1889, while still in the clinic, he painted one of his final self-portraits. In it, we see a somber Van Gogh, painted in a muted light blue. His eyes contain a deep sadness; his expression is heavy. His shoulders slump forward slightly—a posture of defeat, rather than one of strength or vitality. The painting contains a tangible sense of melancholy.

Van Gogh suffered a severe relapse in the asylum from February of 1890 to April of 1890. Shortly after, in May of 1890, he painted *Sorrowing Old Man ("At Eternity's Gate")*. In this piece, an old man sits in a wooden chair, hunched over with his head in his clenched fists, and his elbows resting on his knees. He wears all blue and sits next to a fire. We cannot see his face, only the balding top of his head. The painting is a powerful depiction of sorrow; the old man's suffering is almost palpable.

Shortly after painting *Sorrowing Old Man ("At Eternity's Gate")*, Van Gogh left the clinic and entered the care of Dr. Paul Gachet, who was his physician during the final months of Van Gogh's life. In letters to Theo, Van Gogh spoke highly of Dr. Gachet, but his artwork suggests that he did not feel so positively about Dr. Gachet's ability to help him. In June of 1890, Van Gogh painted *Portrait of Dr. Gachet*. In this piece, Dr. Gachet rests his head in his right hand, his elbow on a red table, alongside two yellow books and a purple foxglove plant. The doctor wears a dark jacket that matches the dark blue background of the painting. His expression is deeply sad and troubled. He looks as if he has given up. The tone is overwhelmingly melancholy.

Remember—this is Van Gogh's depiction of the man who is meant to help him with his emotional and mental difficulties. Van Gogh does not paint a strong, dependable, encouraging doctor who will restore his health. Instead, he paints a slumped over man in total despair, a man who has given up. We do not know if Dr. Gachet was truly at a loss and unable to help Van Gogh or if the defeated image in *Portrait of Dr. Gachet* is Van Gogh's distorted perception of him, but what is clear is that Van Gogh did not see hope for himself even in his own doctor.

In July of 1890, he painted *Wheatfield with Crows*, which some say was his last painting before his death, though this point remains uncertain. The painting shows a dark, ominous sky with clouds moving in. Below the sky is a windswept wheat field, with a deserted path wandering down its center. Crows, often a symbol of death, fly haphazardly above the field. The painting is filled with thick, angry brush strokes. This does not look like a wheat field that one would like to visit; it looks like a scary place where bad things happen. The painting has a powerful feeling of isolation, despair, and impending threat. On July 27, 1890, not long after he painted *Wheatfield with Crows*, it is believed that Van Gogh shot himself in the chest. He died twenty-nine hours later.

To the best of our knowledge, Van Gogh did not experience a singular traumatic event that precipitated his despair, nor did he lack familial support. Rather, an unspecified, serious mental illness was insufficiently treated, and art became his emotional outlet. The emotional threads between his paintings now create a story that we, as viewers, can read—a story of internal distortions, emotional pain, and mental illness. We can see the downward spiral that leads up to his suicide in his artwork.

Magritte, Artemisia, O'Keeffe, Schiele, and Van Gogh are all examples of how our life experience can impact our artistic creations. Magritte experienced a significant trauma that he did not sufficiently process, and his repressed emotions filtered into his creations. Artemisia was assaulted and betrayed by men, which resulted in a focus on women and violence in her art. O'Keeffe was determined to show the world that she could succeed as a female artist, and so she unconsciously infused femininity into her artistic creations. In Schiele's case, the loss of his father and the hypocritical culture in which he grew up influenced his perspective, which is then reflected in the narrow focus and preoccupation in his artwork. Finally, Van Gogh suffered from a mental illness that is expressed in his art. None of these factors—Magritte's childhood trauma, Artemisia's sexual trauma, O'Keeffe's feminist views, Schiele's hypocritical environment, or Van Gogh's mental illness—caused their creative talents; their talents and skills existed independently of these factors. But their unconscious minds did, to varying degrees, shape their art, and thus, fortunately for us, allow us a relatively easy access channel to their unconscious. Their past experiences, attitudes, and emotions filtered into their artwork. We, as viewers, can then interpret the hidden clues within their artwork to gain insight into their minds. You may also gain information about your own unconscious mind if any of these paintings particularly speak to you; I will discuss this concept in depth in Chapter Five.

I hope that the stories of Magritte, Artemisia, O'Keeffe, Schiele, and Van Gogh illustrate the importance of examining our own unconscious minds. That which we are unaware of continues to influence our thoughts, behaviors, and emotions. When left unexamined, these unconscious processes are free to drive our lives and narrow our options and opportunities. We lose sight of many available options. Therefore, it serves our best interest to explore and understand our own motivational unconscious processes. In doing so, we gain insight into the root of our emotion and an understanding of how our perceptions distort reality and influence our behaviors.

While we used to believe that such access to our unconscious was possible only through sophisticated psychotherapeutic explorative techniques, we now know better. Here I propose five channels—memes, slips, artwork, expressive writing, and dreams—to help guide you in this journey of self-exploration. The understanding you gain will provide you with the power to make different choices in life. Had Magritte undertaken this task, perhaps he would have understood how the repressed emotions surrounding his mother's death influenced his artwork. This understanding may then have allowed his emotional wounds to heal, freeing him from the fixation on violent images that he later regretted and perhaps allowing him to find different and happier forms of creation.

The examples of these five artists may be extreme, but we all have unconscious processes that influence our behaviors, perspectives, and emotional reactions. If we want to understand what drives us, why we react the way that we do, why we do what we do, and, in short, what makes us tick, we must delve into our unconscious. Doing so can unearth a wealth of self-knowledge, creative potential, and opportunity for change. It is the goal of this book to help you to embark on this journey, ultimately expanding your creativity, wellness, and self-knowledge.

CHAPTER TWO

Neuroscience of the mind

Research in neuroscience has greatly contributed to our understanding of the mind and brain. We now know a great deal more than in Sigmund Freud's time, though in truth, many aspects of consciousness and the unconscious remain a mystery. Opinions on the neurological basis of consciousness vary widely, from Francis Crick and Christof Koch's theory that consciousness is localized to a specific, small part of the brain called the claustrum, to Gerald Edelman's proposal that consciousness is distributed across the entire brain and that all neurons participate. In fact, consciousness is still an area of active debate (see Carroll, 2016 and Strawson, 2016). The full story of how the mind neurologically functions and produces consciousness will likely not be understood for another fifty to 200 years. However, despite these current limitations in knowledge, the extremely complicated neurological story of the mind is beginning to unfold, providing exciting insight into how different cognitive and emotional processes are formed and controlled.

The biopsychosocial model used in modern day psychiatry proposes that psychological functioning is influenced by biological, psychological, and social factors. As depicted in the figure above, each of these factors interacts with and influences the others to produce both normal and pathological functioning. In bottom-up causation, the neurological processes of the brain, which are the biological factors in this model, produce the mind in all of its various domains of functioning, such as consciousness, thought, and memory. The brain and mind then influence the social context that they operate within.

Developmental psychiatry: culture, mind and brain

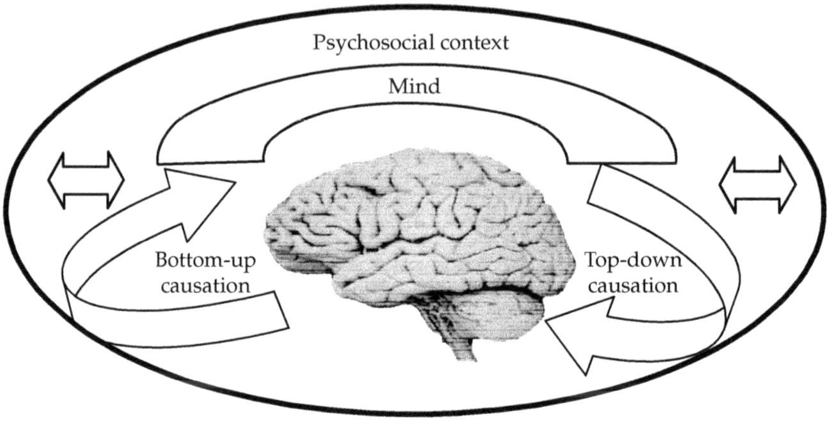

What we have learned most recently, however, is that a second direction influences in this model, a top-down causation, where the mind influences the brain and the social environment influences the mind and brain. At the same time that the neurological functions of the brain produce the processes of the mind, the mind can causally influence the neurological functions of the brain. Processes that occur in the mind can affect how the brain functions neurologically. This is the top-down causation referred to in the figure above. For example, obsessive compulsive disorder (OCD), a disorder in which patients perform rituals to relieve their fears, thoughts, and urges, has been associated with a specific neurological pattern of activity. Theoretically, these neurological processes produce the anxiety and thoughts that plague patients with OCD. However, the symptoms of OCD can be ameliorated with behavioral therapy, in which patients are taught to use willful and conscious efforts to change their problematic behaviors and thoughts, consequently decreasing the associated anxiety. In this treatment, the mind influences the brain. Likewise, the symptoms of Tourette's disorder, a condition in which patients suffer from chronic motor and vocal tics, are caused by neurological abnormalities but can be abated by behavioral therapy. Both of these disorders are examples of top-down causation, in which the mind influences brain processes and functioning, not just in the short run, but also over long periods of time, perhaps even permanently.

The third layer of influence in this model is composed of social factors, such as culture, which can shape and influence both the mind and the brain in top-down causation. Linguistics provides a good example of this phenomenon. Research has shown that learning a second language causes a specific pattern of structural changes in the brain, demonstrating how learned experience can influence neurological development. Similarly, we have known for many decades that the cortical representation of hands is very different in musicians than in non-musicians. Those who use their hands significantly more often and in many more sophisticated ways than in everyday life, such as musicians, develop certain brain patterns which occupy much larger regions in the brain than the rest of us. The brain, mind, and social factors all interact and influence each other, forming a whole that only should be separated for the purpose of scientific inquiry.

Levels of abstraction in normal psychological functioning and psychopathology

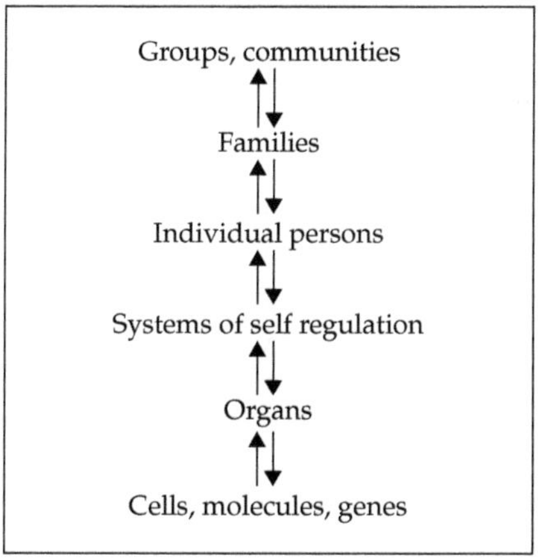

Because functioning is influenced by biological, psychological, and social factors, we can approach the understanding of normal and pathological psychological functioning from different levels of abstraction, from culture to genes, as depicted in the figure above. At the broadest level, problems can be understood by looking at the level of groups and communities. Using this approach, when trying to understand teen drug use, for example, we would consider the role that peer groups and peer pressure have on the problem. At the personal level, this problem would be formulated as a problem with "craving" substances to abuse. At the genetic level we would construct a model that accounts for substance dependence on the basis of a genetic defect, which makes a person more likely to become addicted to certain substances. At the present time and given the state of our knowledge, it is impossible to assign a primary role to any of these models—all should be considered. In fact, it may be possible that there are different forms of drug use that have different causal models supporting them.

Moving proximally within the spheres of social influence, issues in functioning can be approached from the level of the family. Sometimes, behavioral tendencies, such as how we approach conflict, are transgenerational; they are passed on from one generation to the next through social learning. If our parents model anger as a reaction to conflict throughout our childhood, we may then respond to conflict in our own lives with anger through the process of social learning or modeling. Children's learning is powerfully determined by what their parents do, not just what they say. The pattern of troublesome behavior repeats itself in each generation as a result of this transgenerational transmission of attitudes and beliefs. Understanding familial influences can therefore provide insight into understanding an individual's psychology. Memes are a concrete example of a family's operating principles, which influence and shape the way we behave and what we believe. They will be discussed in detail in Chapter Four. Most of us are not aware all the time of what our parents thought the essential rules of life are. To remember, record, and contemplate them, and our reactions to them (whether we have integrated or rejected them) is the first and usually easiest access to our unconscious.

Family environments, of course, do not operate in a biological vacuum. They combine their influences with genes to produce different outcomes. Attention-deficit/hyperactivity disorder (ADHD), which tends to run in families, can be approached in part from the level of familial influence. There most likely is a critical period, during which brain systems mature and come online, and which enable a child to focus and be attentive. This process begins probably in the preschool years and approaches maturation in adolescence. If a child is raised in a chaotic, threatening, unstructured environment, her behavior could evolve into some form of attention dysregulation, especially if she has a genetic loading or predisposition for attention problems. This is an example of how family environment interacts with genes to produce negative outcomes. A structured, calming, supportive family might moderate the influence of the same set of genes considerably. We will give readers a relatively simple but informative model to examine their biological endowment when we discuss our heart rate exercise in combination with the results on our psychological screens in Chapter Three.

Psychological functioning can also be explained and described at the level of the individual person. Each of us has certain propensities and tendencies that contribute to normal and pathological functioning. As we seek to understand ourselves and analyze our own psychological functioning, understanding our own behavioral, emotional, and cognitive tendencies can provide valuable information. Investigating these individual factors will be the primary focus of this book.

At the next level, functioning can be described by systems of self-regulation, such as how we self-regulate our own negative and positive emotions, cope with stress, and employ different defensive mechanisms. For example, problems with attachment can be understood by looking at anxiety level—people who experience high levels of anxiety tend to have more problems with attachment. Self-regulation systems will be discussed in more detail in Chapter Three.

Moving in one notch from systems of self-regulation, problems in functioning can be described in terms of organ dysfunction. For example, the inability to express abstract concepts is associated with abnormalities in temporal lobe functioning, which is a specific area of the brain. Finally, normal and pathological functioning can sometimes be reduced to the level of cells, molecules, and genes. Huntington's disease, an inherited neurological disease that causes motor, emotional, and cognitive impairments, results from a single abnormal gene.

An important point to remember when considering these different levels is that not every problem can be reduced to each level of abstraction, and each level of abstraction cannot necessarily be reduced to a lower level. An individual problem with anger management may be better understood at the familial and individual level than at the level of organ dysfunction. Similarly, a problem that occurs at the individual level may not be reducible to a genetic abnormality. Genetic and molecular facts need to be embedded within the larger psychosocial context in order to understand the whole picture of pathology and wellness.

Although neuroscience is only one piece of the puzzle in understanding how we function, it is nonetheless an important field that has made significant contributions to our understanding of human functioning. Before delving into the nitty gritty of neuroscientific research, let's go over some basic neurobiology, or anatomy of the brain. Using imaging technologies, scientists have mapped the brain into discrete regions that are associated with different functions. For the purposes of this book, the brain can be functionally divided into two sections: the limbic system, which is the inner layer of the brain, and the cerebral cortex, which is the outermost layer of brain tissue. Each of these areas is then subdivided into more specific brain regions that control distinct processes. The limbic system can be seen as the system for emotional activation—an emotional gas pedal—among other functions. The cortex, particularly the frontal and parietal cortex, acts as a brake pedal. In close proximity to the limbic system are structures that are important in memory formation, such as the hippocampus and the amygdala. Memory formation and how it is related to emotions will be discussed in detail later in this chapter.

In addition to the limbic system and the cerebral cortex, there are many other important regions in the brain, such as the cerebellum, which by and large contributes to our locomotion. As we are not looking into locomotive processes of humans here, we will not concern ourselves with the cerebellum and related structures extensively.

The brain structures that collectively compose the limbic system are the thalamus, cingulate gyrus, fornix, amygdala, hippocampus, and parahippocampal gyrus. These regions, considered to be the more evolutionary primitive areas of the brain, are present in a wide range of species, including reptiles.

An important function of the limbic system is to produce emotions. While humans experience a wide range of different emotions, many researchers agree that there are six basic emotions that are hardwired within the limbic system: anger, sadness, fear, disgust, happiness, and surprise. Imaging techniques have been used to locate the neurological structures and pathways associated with some of these basic emotions, such as fear, with reasonable accuracy. The ability to locate these emotions neurologically highlights their universal nature. Evolutionarily, it makes sense that the emotions crucial to survival, such as fear, would be so rigidly hardwired in the brain.

As we mature and neurologically develop, we gain more complex emotions, such as shame, contempt, admiration, and guilt, which have a large experiential and learned component. Rather than being hardwired, we must learn these emotions under the impact of social modeling and experience. They involve multiple interacting structures and pathways in the brain and are very difficult to locate neurologically using imaging studies. As we develop, our emotions branch like a tree into increasingly complex and differentiated entities, which are correspondingly more difficult to assign to a specific locus. This fact accounts for much of the uncertainty and contradictions in neuroscientific and psychological research. As we go up the ladder of complexity, we struggle with certainty, reliability, and sometimes even validity. All this amounts to is that we are dealing with very complicated structures which are not easily understood by the classical scientific methods that often rely on reduction to the simplest elements as we are trying to understand the nature and function of such complicated entities like motives, emotions, impulse control, and personalities.

By producing emotions, the limbic system is in turn responsible for producing emotionally driven behaviors, such as fleeing from a predator in response to fear. Finally, the limbic system drives instinctual behaviors which, like emotionally driven behaviors, do not require conscious thought. This portion of the brain is responsible for decreasing energy expenditure when an animal is tired, eating when it feels hungry, and drinking when it feels thirsty.

The neurological structures that make up the cerebral cortex are the frontal lobe, parietal lobe, temporal lobe, and occipital lobe. They are considered more recent evolutionary developments of the brain than the limbic system, containing literally billions of neurons that are interconnected in ways which we are just beginning to understand. The myriads of ways of interconnectedness and the sheer number of neurons give rise to a complexity of functions that are unique in the universe and most likely account for much of the highest functions in humans. The cerebral cortex is responsible for sophisticated cognitive functions, such as consciousness, attention, thought, and language. While other species do have a cerebral cortex, the capabilities of the human cerebral cortex are significantly more complex and extensive. Another characteristic that emerges from this complicated network is our human capacity for flexibility in thought and action and the complexity of aspects that form ourselves. This highest form of achievement is the most likely reason why we are so successful as a species—in the Darwinian sense. It is the bane of the mental health sciences because it makes the life of a researcher and clinician so difficult. The answer to the question, "Why did Magritte or O'Keeffe paint what and in the way they did?" is never simple. It arises out of a complex set of interactions with the piece of art, our own selves, and our history.

The cerebral cortex and the limbic system are in constant interplay. If the limbic system is the brain's emotional gas pedal, the cerebral cortex acts as its brake pedal, regulating and controlling the instincts, impulses, and emotions produced by the limbic system. Have you ever been on a diet and successfully resisted eating that hamburger, no matter how hungry you felt? That triumph was possible thanks to your cerebral cortex, which exerted conscious regulatory processes over your behavior, despite your limbic system's instinctual impulse to eat. Likewise, any of us who has been on a diet knows that sometimes we just can't resist that hamburger. In these instances, the limbic system wins the battle.

Similarly, the cerebral cortex serves to regulate and control, or at least rein in, our wide range of emotions and resulting behaviors. Consider the difference in emotional expression and regulation between a lion and a person. If we were to provoke a lion, it would instinctively display aggressive behaviors toward us, and, given the chance, it would likely act on those aggressive instincts, much to our dismay. A lion does not consciously stop itself from attacking; it simply experiences the emotion and acts on it. Humans are capable of a much greater degree of control over their response to anger. We can consciously control our behavioral responses to emotions, giving us the power to choose from a variety of reactions in response to feeling angry, from getting into a fistfight to walking away. This power reflects the regulatory abilities of the human cerebral cortex on the limbic system. Given time, work space, and the right tools, such as reflection, self-observation, and the capacity to retain and consider a social code of action, we can make prudent and adaptive choices. This assumption is very strong in the depth psychologies and provides the main rationale for making the unconscious conscious. It does of course not mean that all of us will do so at all times and in all circumstances.

We do not always cognitively regulate and control emotional responses. Sometimes we employ an alternative, more primitive neurological emotional response pathway that does not require cognitive processing. This pathway is called the emotional brain, a term coined by Joseph LeDoux (2000, 2003) to describe the circuit in the brain that produces instinctive emotional responses. Most of the research on the emotional brain is centered on the amygdala, which is a part of the limbic system, the driver of emotions and emotional responses. The amygdala is specifically responsible for the learning and expression of fear responses.

Let's look at an example of how the emotional brain works to produce a fear response. Have you ever been startled by something, without even realizing what startled you until after you had already jumped? Perhaps you were going for a walk in the woods, and suddenly you jumped. It was not until after you had reacted that you realized you thought you had seen a snake, which in actual fact was just a twig. You did not see the "snake," feel scared, cognitively assess the situation, and then plan a response. Rather, you instinctively and instantly responded to the stimulus before you even recognized it. In the instant that you jumped, you did not recognize what was happening or why. Your conscious experience of fear came after you responded instinctively and emotionally. You activated what LeDoux calls "the low road" of anxious experience, which has an important protective function for us when there is potential danger and not a lot of time to think.

When the emotional brain circuit is activated, the emotional response to a stimulus occurs unconsciously and without cognitive involvement. The sensory thalamus recognizes the emotional stimulus, such as the possible snake, and sends this signal to the amygdala, which then orchestrates the emotional response by sending signals to the behavioral, autonomic, and endocrine response control systems in the brain stem. This pathway bypasses the cerebral cortex and causes a reaction without any conscious thought. Only after we react to the threat do we assess the situation and consciously realize that we are scared.

The evolutionary purpose of this neurological circuit is probably to save time when responding to threats. If we cognitively assessed every situation before reacting to it, we would take much longer to respond to a threat. That snake would probably have already attacked us while we were busy thinking about how to react. Bypassing the cerebral cortex decreases reaction time and improves survival when reacting rapidly is of the essence.

Emotional responses are therefore quite necessary for survival. Emotions are the guiding force when it comes to navigating both environmental dangers and social interactions. Researchers have used animal studies to knock out the limbic system, rendering the animals emotionally incapable. The primary result of this neural manipulation is simple—the animals die rapidly, even in a protected laboratory environment. If we think through the consequences of shutting down emotions, it comes as no surprise that survival is significantly compromised. Imagine an animal with no ability to feel fear or anger. When a gazelle is drinking at a water hole, how would it know to immediately flee when a lion approaches, if it feels absolutely no fear of the lion? Similarly, what would motivate an animal to fight back when it is attacked if it is incapable of feeling anger? Emotions serve the same kind of behavioral guidance in humans. As much as we may consider emotions like fear and aggression unpleasant elements of life, they have important functions. Our emotions are in a state of constant ebb and flow as we move through our daily lives. They are like a compass that guides us in the daily traffic of human interactions. If we are oblivious to them, we would probably not be as successful in staying out of trouble or finding fulfillment and happiness as we go about the business of daily living.

In order to be able to be guided by our emotions and learn from them, we must be able to recognize and distinguish different emotions, both in ourselves and in others. Of all the different ways we communicate emotional states to each other, such as vocalizations, body language, and gestures, facial expressions are by far the most expressive tool according to research. Charles Darwin was the first to recognize that some emotions are ubiquitous and universally recognized, as he detailed in his 1872 publication *The Expression of Emotions in Man and Animals*. Just as Darwin proposed, evidence has since shown that facial expressions not only communicate the greatest diversity of emotions, but that those related to the six basic emotions are universal in humans. People from cultures around the world both utilize and recognize the same facial movements in order to express these emotions, a fact that suggests that this emotional expression and recognition is hard wired, rather than learned. It makes sense evolutionarily, as it would be in our best interest to recognize something like fear in others in order to communicate the presence of a predator, for example. Vocal signals, such as laughing and crying, are also universally recognizable across different cultures. However, the range of emotions communicated by vocal signals is not as large as that of facial expressions.

Correctly identifying emotions in others is an important skill, but correctly identifying our own emotions is arguably even more important. When our hearts start racing, how do we know if it is excitement or fear? In the 1960s, two researchers, Stanley Schachter and Jerome

Singer, investigated how we identify and label our emotions. They hypothesized that we use a combination of both internal and external cues to label and identify an emotion. Internal cues refer to the physical symptoms of physiological arousal, such as a pounding heart or sweaty palms. External cues refer to the cognitive processes of interpreting the environment and deciphering a feeling based on the circumstances of the given situation.

Before Schachter and Singer's study, researchers had found that many different emotions, from fear to excitement, were associated with the same physical sensations, such as a pounding heart, suggesting that we do not use internal cues alone to identify emotions. It remains an open question whether emotions are this undifferentiated at the physiological level, as these results have not been replicated. However, the suggestion that many different emotions have the same physiological pattern led Schachter and Singer to hypothesize that emotional identification is a biopsychosocial process, rather than a strictly biological process, and involves both internal and external cues.

In their study, they found that physiological arousal is necessary but not sufficient to produce the conscious experience of an emotion. Participants put in situations expected to induce an emotion, but who felt no physical symptoms of arousal, were less likely to report experiencing an emotion than those who did have symptoms. The finding suggests that physiological arousal is a necessary condition for a conscious emotional experience to occur and that cognitive factors alone are not always sufficient. Walking down a dark alley and cognitively determining it to be dangerous without any physical feeling of fear, like a pounding heart, would likely not be reported as a scary experience.

Physiological symptoms alone were also not sufficient to induce an emotion. Subjects who had a logical explanation for their physiological arousal were less likely to identify the feeling as an emotion than those that did not. We can notice the physical sensations often associated with emotions without labeling the experience as an emotional one, suggesting that physiological arousal is only part of the puzzle when it comes to emotional experiences. If our hearts were to start pounding and we knew that we had just had a large caffeinated coffee, we would likely interpret the physical sensation of a pounding heart as a side effect of the caffeine, rather than as an emotion.

In reality, identifying and labeling emotions is dependent on the interaction between both internal physical sensations and external cognitive factors. When an event arouses the sympathetic nervous system, the context of the event, as well as past experience, is used to label that feeling. Walking down that dark alley, we might start to feel our hearts pounding, a sensation we could interpret as many different emotions. We would then use cognitive cues to determine that it is fear we feel, perhaps remembering that a friend had been mugged in an alley, and that this is therefore a dangerous situation. If, on the other hand, we were on a first date when we felt our hearts pounding, we would be more likely to use cognitive cues to interpret the feeling as excitement. Both sympathetic arousal and cognitive processes are necessary for conscious emotional states to occur.

Some emotions are more contextual than others and require a certain amount of ongoing heuristic interpretation. In this process, we interpret our physiological state in light of social context. The dependence of these emotions on interpretative processes opens the door for misinterpretation. Unconscious defensiveness can influence and distort how we interpret situations and consciously experience emotions. Consequently, we do not always correctly identify our emotions. I will discuss defenses in detail in Chapter Three.

A patient of mine whose father unexpectedly passed away exemplifies how defensive processes can influence emotional identification. Since his death, she had avoided expressing her own grief for fear of further upsetting her grieving mother. She came to see me on the anniversary of her father's death. Despite the heavy emotions I expected her to feel on this day, she insisted that she felt fine. Although she continued to deny any feelings of distress, she did report unusual physical sensations, such as an increased heart rate, wet palms, pressure behind her eyes, dry mouth, feelings of restlessness, and a lump in her throat. Based on the context, I interpreted these physical feelings as symptoms of distress and grief over the loss of her father. She wanted no part of that. I knew her father had been very dear and important to her. By dissembling the emotion of sadness and fear and reducing it to its bare biological constituents, she spared her mother and herself the return of grief at the loss of this important person. By focusing on the physiological manifestations of the emotion without the heuristic process of cognitive interpretation, she reduced the emotion to its various physical components in an effort to control it. Her fear of burdening her mother was so strong that she misinterpreted her own feelings and was unable to identify her emotions correctly. This case underscores how unconscious defensive processes can affect emotional identification (the correct label for this process in classical defense parlance would be somatization).

In addition to the neurological basis of emotions, interesting advances have been made in the study of memory processes. Memories are broadly divided into two categories—procedural and declarative. Procedural, or implicit, memory is the unconscious memory we use for perceptual and motor skills. This is the memory that allows us to wake up each day remembering how to walk or ride a bike, without much, if any, effort. Procedural memory involves the cerebellum, striatum, amygdala, and sensory and motor pathways.

Declarative, or explicit, memory involves the conscious recall of information about people, places, and things, such as someone's name. These processes take place in the medial temporal lobe and, in particular, in the hippocampus. Episodic memory is a specific type of declarative memory that refers to the memory of autobiographical information and emotionally charged events, like remembering a wedding day. In contrast to other types of memory, episodic memories are uniquely time stamped—we remember when these emotional events occurred. These memories hang around in our unconscious and influence how we live our lives. This is especially evident when we approach significant anniversaries, such as wedding days, death days, and commemorations of big historical events. We may feel an increasing sense of happiness, sadness, or feelings of threat as the calendar approaches these days without our consciously being aware of what is about to come. Accessing episodic memories therefore plays an important role in accessing the unconscious. Episodic memory is also involved in some psychiatric disturbances, such as post-traumatic stress disorder (PTSD). Reliving the traumatic events involved in PTSD is essentially an extreme form of the return of episodic memory.

Both procedural and declarative memory processes have two different types of storage—short-term memory (lasting minutes to hours), and long-term memory (lasting days, weeks, or longer). According to Eric Kandel's research on the California sea slug, the fact that short-term and long-term memories require different chemicals within the brain indicates that they are neurologically distinct processes.

In order to move information from short-term into long-term storage, we must do three things: sleep, rehearse, and retell. Sleeping is critical to memory storage. When we sleep, we sort through the contents of our short-term memory and decide what to store permanently and what to discard. Evidence of this sorting can be found in dreams, which contain elements of personal experiences and events. In order to solidify the contents of our short-term memory in our long-term memory, we need to rehearse them and retell them in our waking life. The concept is a familiar concept to most of us. When cramming for an exam, for example, we store the information temporarily in short-term memory, and we can regurgitate the information during the exam. If we do not continue to review the information, we find that—despite an A grade—not long after the exam we have forgotten all of the material.

It is plausible that, at any given time, we can only hold so much information in short-term memory before it is either discarded or moved into long-term storage. In contrast, when we have gone over something many times, such as the alphabet, the information or event becomes acquired wisdom and is always accessible. That information has been moved into long-term storage. If an event, experience, or piece of information is undesirable in some way—perhaps it was a traumatic event—we sometimes avoid talking about it, which can impair the long-term storage of the memory.

Working memory is a type of short-term memory that refers to the information that we can pay attention to at any given time. Just like a computer, our capacity for working memory is limited. Studies have shown that on average, we can only hold three to four items, such as digits, letters, or words, in our working memory at one time. When items are grouped together into clusters of three to four, we are able to hold an average of seven units in working memory. Phone numbers consist of seven numbers that are usually clustered into groups of three or four numbers. If our working memories are loaded with irrelevant data, such as unimportant sensory stimuli, our ability to attend to a task at hand is limited. This is one of the problems in disorders such as attention-deficit/hyperactivity disorder (ADHD).

Individual working memory capacities can vary from the average of three to four items. One interesting line of research has examined the relationship between working memory and the tendency to repress intrusive thoughts and unwanted memories. Studies have found that those of us who tend to repress more often have larger than average working memory capacities; likewise, those with greater working memory capacities are better able to suppress thoughts intentionally. The findings make sense: Working memory is defined as the amount of information that we can focus our attention on at one time. In order to control our focus of attention on those three to four items, we must exclude irrelevant material from our consciousness, ignoring unwanted thoughts, memories, and information. In other words, we must repress these unwanted thoughts. This research suggests that working memory and repression may go hand in hand.

Memory, particularly episodic memory, is intimately tied to emotion. A significant amount of memory formation takes place in the limbic system, the region of the brain responsible for emotions. In 1981, Gordon Bower discussed the interplay between emotion and memory by reviewing the evidence that memory is mood-state dependent. Using hypnosis to induce different emotional states in his subjects, Bower demonstrated that memory improved when the mood during the experience or learning event matched the mood during recall. Subjects were also better able to recall more emotionally intense events than less emotionally intense events. So, if we were sitting on the beach, happy as a clam, we would likely be more able to remember happy childhood memories, such as going to Disneyland with our families, than negative ones, such as fighting with siblings. Our ability to remember highly emotionally charged happy memories would be particularly increased there, at the beach.

Bower theorized that memories are filed away in the brain according to emotion, which acts as a memory unit. When an emotion is activated, this activation spreads to the events and concepts that are linked to it, thus aiding the retrieval of the memories associated with this emotion. Picture the brain as a filing cabinet, with each file labeled as a different emotion. Our happiness files contain all of our associations with happiness, including memories of past experiences that we relate to being happy. In this file we might find that trip to Disneyland, winning a soccer game, and opening birthday presents. In order to access any of these happy memories, we must open the happiness file. Opening the file requires activating the brain's happiness node, which can be accomplished by experiencing the emotion. Joyfully sitting on the beach activates happiness within the brain, which unlocks the happiness file, providing access to all those wonderful memories.

Trying to remember these good times would be less successful if we did so while watching a particularly heart-wrenching movie, because by activating the conflicting emotion of sadness, we activate a different set of memories and associations. Opening the brain's sadness file unleashes our collection of sad memories. In the effort to remember a happy childhood event, these sad memories would create interference and decrease our ability to retrieve that memory of Disneyland. This concept has important implications in accessing the motivational unconscious through expressive writing, which will be discussed in Chapter Six.

Emotions not only affect our ability to recall memories, but they also influence which information we focus on during an event and, in turn, which information we remember. In Bower's study, when subjects were exposed to a narrative that matched their mood at the time of learning, they better remembered the events of the narrative. A subject who was angry while reading a narrative paid more attention to the angry characters and remembered more about these characters than happy ones. Emotion contributes to our selection of what we deem important to remember from life. It also can contaminate events as they are being recalled.

Given Bower's findings, we conclude that the best way to remember a past event is to recreate the mental state that we were in during memory formation. However, what about those memories that we would rather forget and, indeed, do successfully forget? Freud was the first to propose that unwanted memories can be repressed into the unconscious, thereby eliminating them from conscious awareness. Recent advances in cognitive neuroscience have begun to identify the neurobiological mechanism of memory repression.

Using functional magnetic resonance imaging (fMRI) of the brain, Michael Anderson and colleagues discovered that the repression of unwanted memories is associated with a particular pattern of brain activity—increased dorsolateral prefrontal activation and decreased hippocampal activation. The hippocampus is an important player in declarative memory formation. When a memory is repressed, the memory retrieval process is in some way inhibited. It makes sense that decreasing the ability to retrieve a memory—memory repression—would involve decreased activity of the brain regions involved in memory formation and retrieval—the hippocampus. But what causes this decreased activity in the hippocampus? Increased dorsolateral prefrontal activation could be the second piece of the puzzle. The lateral prefrontal cortex is associated with stopping motor responses, changing tasks, and overcoming interference during cognitive tasks. Each of these tasks requires suppressing some type of brain activity—stopping a motor response requires suppressing motor pathways; changing tasks requires that attention be moved from one task to another, thus suspending attention to the first task; and overcoming interference similarly requires halting attention to the interfering stimuli. Given these findings, it seems possible that the dorsolateral prefrontal cortex suppresses the hippocampus, thus suppressing memory retrieval and leading to memory repression.

The more we consciously and deliberately suppress the retrieval of a memory, the less able we are to remember it in the future. It may sound redundant that when we repress a memory, we then cannot remember it. However, this finding hints at the important distinction between memory repression and forgetting. When we repress a memory, we actively block memory retrieval. The memory does exist somewhere within our brain and is theoretically retrievable. Conversely, when we have truly forgotten, the memory is no longer stored in our brain and we may not be able to retrieve it, no matter how much we may try. The findings in this study suggest that there is an interaction between the two, in which actively repressing a memory may then cause us to actually forget it. They provide neurobiological evidence that what we forget may give us insight into what we may be unconsciously repressing.

There is another important distinction to make here—the difference between conscious and unconscious memory repression. Conscious memory repression is the process of intentionally trying not to think about unwanted memories. We consciously stop unpleasant memories from entering our awareness. This is the type of memory repression that Anderson and colleagues studied. Therefore the experimental evidence that memory repression is associated with increased dorsolateral prefrontal activation and decreased hippocampal activation is limited specifically to conscious memory repression.

Memory repression can also be an unconscious process that happens automatically and without any conscious intention. In this case, memory repression is a type of unconscious defense mechanism that serves to protect us from the awareness of unpleasant memories.

Studies on dissociative amnesia have begun to provide information about the neurological underpinnings of unconscious memory repression. Patients with dissociative amnesia, a disorder that typically occurs as a result of a traumatic or stressful event, are unable to remember specific, usually negative, memories. No physical cause for their memory impairment is evident, and the disorder is classified as a psychiatric condition whereby the patient unconsciously and automatically employs memory repression as a defense mechanism in order to avoid the emotional trauma caused by an event.

One study showed that the unconscious memory repression associated with dissociative amnesia is linked to decreased hippocampal activity and increased activity in the prefrontal cortex. This neurological pattern is the same one that Anderson's study associated with conscious memory repression. Evidence continues to support the hypothesis that the prefrontal cortex somehow inhibits hippocampal activity, thereby inhibiting memory retrieval and potentially resulting in both conscious and unconscious memory repression.

One of the most interesting advances in neuroscience has been the discovery of the default network, which is the network of brain structures associated with free thinking and internally focused cognitive processes. Researchers were first alerted to the default network by accident while they were investigating the neurological basis of goal-oriented cognitive functions. In these experiments, when an area lit up on a functional magnetic resonance imaging scan (fMRI) while a subject performed a specific task, researchers could conclude that these areas were somehow involved in the cognitive process being tested. As a control to these experimental conditions, subjects were asked not to focus on anything in particular. However, the researchers soon realized that this "rest" state was not as neurologically restful as they had expected. Over and over, they observed that specific areas of the brain were consistently activated when people were left to think quietly to themselves (Buckner, Andrews-Hanna, & Schacter, 2008).

They discovered that the brain is actually quite active during this rest state. In the same way that the motor system or the visual system involves specific brain structures, the default network is an anatomically defined brain system composed of multiple interacting structures. These structures have individually been associated with functions like memory formation, emotions, and self-regulation.

When idle, internally focused cognitive processes are spontaneously and almost immediately engaged, such as remembering past autobiographical information and experiences, as well as envisioning and planning future events. When we have nothing we must focus on, we spontaneously reminisce, reflect, plan, and imagine.

A number of brain systems are active when we rest, from visual to language networks. However, the default network is the only one that is not only active when we rest, but also deactivates during task performance. When we perform an attention demanding cognitive task, for example, our default network activity subsides. When we finish the task and our brains are left idle, the default network comes back into play. It can also be preferentially activated during a few specific tasks, such as retrieving an episodic memory, planning or imagining a future event, self-judgment tasks, envisioning the beliefs of another person (theory of mind), and moral decision-making.

Most of us are familiar with this phenomenon. How often have you found yourself daydreaming about possible future events, replaying past conversations, or rehearsing future interactions? Most of have thoughts like these all the time. Our heads are often filled with internal monologues and vivid imagery. Without an external task to focus on, our minds wander, not into ordered thought, but into a stream of consciousness. We daydream, fantasize, imagine, and think about ourselves quite avidly. In fact, 96 percent of people report daydreaming every day. Rather than intentionally planning to sit down and think these things, our brains seem to engage the default network and conjure these thoughts automatically and unconsciously (Koch, 2012).

The default network is most active when we are at rest, and its activity tends to decrease when we must focus on an external task. This suggests that there is competition between internally and externally focused cognition for a limited amount of brain energy. Focusing attention on external tasks and information decreases our ability to focus internally, and vice versa. Again, we are familiar with the pattern. When you are at work and you begin to daydream, does your productivity increase or decrease? Daydreaming typically interferes with our ability to pay attention to demanding tasks at hand.

By the same token, if the goal were to access this internal mode of cognition, eliminating external distractions and tasks would maximize the chances of being able to do so. I see this in clinical practice regularly: The patient who engages in an external task during psychotherapy has a difficult time accessing the internal thoughts and emotions that need attention. I once worked with a child who always wanted to play board games during our sessions. The board game allowed her to divert her attention away from the scary emotional topics that she was there to work through. This is the basis behind the traditionally simplistic couch and chair setup of psychotherapy offices—minimizing external stimuli fosters maximal internal reflection.

What purpose would it serve us to think spontaneously about ourselves, our pasts, and our futures whenever we are not otherwise engaged? One hypothesis is that the thoughts produced by the default network during rest allow us to plan for future events. Autobiographical memory and theory of mind are important elements of this process. When planning for a job interview, we may think about the last interview we had and how we can improve our chances of success. Understanding why we did not get the first job would require us to replay the interview (autobiographical memory), think about how the interviewer perceived our responses, and process why he believed we were not right for the job (theory of mind). In doing so, we better prepare ourselves for the next interview.

Biographical narratives also provide a work space to emotionally process important events and memories, a concept that will be covered in greater detail in Chapter Six when I discuss expressive writing. Likewise, understanding the mental landscape of other people is a skill that will be put to use in Chapter Five in order to conceive the emotions behind artwork and the artist's intent.

By replaying past experiences, going over past social interactions, thinking about how other people reacted and felt, and constructing different simulations, we can improve our planning for future events and navigate social interactions. We utilize otherwise unproductive downtime to learn from our past experiences and create predictions about upcoming events. According to this explanation, the free thinking produced by the default network is a healthy and adaptive process.

The default network is what we try to activate when we want to access the motivational unconscious. This is not accomplished by following logical, rational thoughts such as "My name is Hans. I am from Austria. I am a psychiatrist." Though these are accurate autobiographical details, they do not reveal any information about my underlying thoughts, feelings, or beliefs. Instead, it is my internally focused, emotionally driven stream of consciousness produced by my own default network that will reveal my unconscious thoughts and emotions. Asking me, for instance, about my reasons for emigrating to the United States would most likely set my own default network ablaze with activity. This decision clearly was and is very emotionally charged, and even after many years of thinking about it, I am not sure I fully understand it.

Our default network can link us to the emotions and thoughts simmering below the surface that we may not even have been aware of. To access our unconscious, we must pay attention to where our minds wander and follow our emotional rivers, allowing ourselves to free-associate thoughts based on emotional links. Engaging the default network and following the emotional tone of thoughts and behaviors are the keys to accessing the unconscious. I will provide many examples of what this process looks like in Chapters Four to Seven. More information about the default network, including images of brain scans, can be found by searching "default network" on the web.

A final word on the progress in the neurosciences that we can expect over the next decade in this area of study: Under the influence of the "decade of the brain," which has accelerated our knowledge in any of the areas discussed in this chapter vastly, we can expect that much more science will become relevant to this context. To be fair, it is also true that it is very hard for the layman, and I have to say also the professional, to keep abreast of all the developments. We have tried very hard to strike a satisfactory balance between what is known now, what has been known for some time, and where the field is most likely moving to in the future. Very often, some of our younger scientists remark that they see no particular reason to quote Sigmund Freud and all his mistakes. I usually reply that for all his mistakes he also had an amazing number of brilliant insights which neuroscience has confirmed (for instance, much of his thinking about the tripartite structure of the brain, where he anticipated many of neuroscience's findings over 100 years later). I also say that mental health knowledge is not based on neuroscience alone, it is also based on our knowledge of people. That of course is also risky for different reasons. But in sum total, we have to respect both of these sources of information as we try to understand ourselves better. And then I say, with a smile: for every patient that gives me wrong ideas, you neuroscientists have a paper which will be either rejected or never read again in three or four years—because that is the current half-life of medical information in this field.

CHAPTER THREE

The role of psychometrics in the study of the unconscious: what are your personal preferences in resolving stress, conflict, and ambiguity?

Screening your personality: the GHQ-30, FAY, WAI-84, heart rate exercise, and REM-71

Neuroscience research has considerably advanced mental health knowledge, but it is only half of the story. We need to be able to apply the insights of neuroscience to the individual. "Amygdala controls" and "frontal lobe controls" need to be translated into concepts that are applicable to our own personal experience. One other important source of information comes into play here: clinical practice—what mental health professionals have observed in the course of studying actual human behavior. These insights have led to practices and tools that aid in understanding the unconscious and the barriers to bringing it into consciousness.

Many, but not all, psychologists and psychiatrists are professionally trained in how to access and evaluate the motivational unconscious. This skill of learning how to read people involves interpreting both verbal and nonverbal cues in a manner that penetrates below the surface level of the conscious mind. Much of how we perceive the world and how we behave is driven by emotion rather than logic. Reading people requires paying attention to the emotional undertones of speech, behavior, and facial expressions, rather than listening to what an individual may actually be saying. For example, has anyone ever told you that he is not angry with you, but his behavior, however subtle, suggests otherwise?

His eye slits may narrow, his brow furrows, perhaps he is tapping his feet or clenching his fists.

In this way we may consciously believe and express one idea—that we are not angry—but our emotions in the unconscious mind produce conflicting nonverbal cues. Facial expressions are a good indicator of this phenomenon. While we have conscious control over our choice of words, we are usually unaware of the small changes in our facial expression and body language. These changes reflect fleeting unconscious emotional processes, sometimes only microseconds long. Emotion is the bridge that links the conscious and unconscious mind. By following these emotional patterns, we learn the truth within the motivational unconscious.

In the previous chapter, I discussed how emotions, beliefs, and attitudes affect our memories and what we pay attention to. I know this neuroscience discussion is dense and taxing, so let me recapitulate.

Our unconscious mind determines how we experience and remember an event. During an experience, which elements of the event we focus on is partially controlled by emotion. Each of us will choose different pieces of the environment and events to pay attention to and remember. Though we each differ significantly in the information we select as important, what each one of us focuses on in different situations remains fairly constant. In different situations, we each tend to pay attention to the same types of things. This selection process is driven by both emotion and other traits, such as conscious and unconscious self-regulation. Traits differ from acute states; they are tendencies that extend over time. It is also important to remember that with effort, we can override whatever traits and propensities we have. The emphasis here is on effort—we need to expend energy to do this. This type of flexibility is what makes us human—we are not simple robots who behave the same way every time we are up against a challenge. That would not make us very successful in terms of adaptation. But if left to our own devices, we do have a certain tendency—a probabilistic way of responding—that can be measured and known.

What we remember of experiences, and indeed if we remember them at all, is also dictated unconsciously by our emotions. We do not decide what to remember; rather, the emotional charge of an event triggers the memory formation. This is why we can remember intimate details of highly emotional events, such as the birth of a child ten years ago, but we may not remember what we had for lunch yesterday.

Emotions, consequently, determine what we pay attention to, what we remember, and how we remember it. These processes take place automatically and unconsciously. By following the emotional stream within speech, behavior, and memories, rather than paying attention to rational logic, psychiatrists can gain access to the unconscious processes that shape our behavior. Each of us can also gain insight into our own motivational unconscious by paying attention to our emotional instincts and patterns in the same manner.

Another tool I utilize to gain information about the motivational unconscious is psychological questionnaires, called psychometrics. The screens and tests we will introduce you to in this chapter allow for flexibility and range of responses. They do not measure mental disorders or assign you a diagnosis. They measure normative behavior, emotions, and attitudes, that is, a range of possible responses found in all humans. These responses usually change as we age or as we get stressed and upset. They can also change if we are in some form of therapy, usually not dramatically, but more as a matter of degree. These tests do not deliver certainty, but rather probability. And they all stand in some relationship—either facilitative or impeding—to the exercises we will ask you to do in this book to access your secret mind. We have tested these influences in many of our students and have found moderate, but consistent, relationships. The purpose of giving you these tests to complete is to prepare you for what you are about to encounter as you are trying to get in touch with your unconscious.

These questionnaires provide an analysis of adaptive styles and dispositions by assessing our emotional landscape and patterns of self-regulation. Self-regulation, or emotional regulation, has emerged in the past decade or two as an area of great interest in psychology. One of the most prominent and active researchers in the field is one of my colleagues here at Stanford, James Gross, Ph.D. He has written extensively on this subject (see Gross, 2009). Self-regulation refers to our tendency to keep emotions and behavior under control in even the most stressful circumstances. Self-regulation processes can be divided into consciously steered efforts and automatic, unconscious tendencies. Freudian language calls the latter processes "defenses." Repression is a very well-known and recognized defense, as is denial. Self-regulation is a more encompassing term, as it also refers to the control of one's environment in the effort to keep things on an even keel. Freudian defenses usually refer to internal processes.

Most of us experience the same wide range of emotions, but to varying degrees. The questionnaires assess how much we experience different positive and negative emotions. We also differ in how much we consciously self-regulate our emotions and behavior. One prominent label for this type of self-regulation is *restraint*. Similarly, we all exhibit different degrees of unconscious repression, minimization, and denial of our negative emotions and thoughts. Psychometric tests analyze this level of repression, providing information about the difficulty we have in delving into our unconscious minds.

Finally, as we discussed above, defenses are reflexive, rapid ways of explaining to ourselves why certain things keep happening to us. They shield us from difficult things that we do not want to think about. Each of us has different habitual defenses that we automatically use when we do not want to pay attention to a distressing emotion, event, or impulse. These defenses can distort our perception of reality and prevent us from learning new information about the world and ourselves. Psychometric tests provide a profile of the defenses we favor and, consequently, of how these unconscious processes affect our perceptions and interpretations of reality. Some defenses can pose more of an obstacle than others to doing the exercises in Chapters Four to Seven. Defenses will be discussed in greater depth later in this chapter as part of the description of the Response Evaluation Measure (REM-71). Understanding what defenses we most often utilize, how we cope under adverse circumstances, and how much we repress or deny negative emotions allows psychiatrists to better determine how to access our motivational unconscious (Huemer et al., 2015).

In the rest of this chapter, I will provide an overview of four psychometric questionnaires—the General Health Questionnaire (GHQ), Facts About You (FAY), the Weinberger Adjustment Inventory (WAI), and the Response Evaluation Measure (REM). Each of these has demonstrated validity, the degree to which a measure represents the intended construct, and reliability, the consistency of scores between assessments. We have used these instruments for many years in our studies, in the classes I have taught, and in my clinical practice. We have also been able to study them in relationship to the types of exercises we are introducing you to. The questionnaires provide an important first step as you prepare to enter into your secret mind.

The Appendix at the end of this book provides most of these questionnaires for you to copy and fill out for your personal use. For the GHQ-30, information is provided on how to obtain the screen online. The Appendix also provides scoring instructions and norms, which help you to interpret your results.

The General Health Questionnaire (GHQ)

The first psychometric measure that can be used to gain a baseline understanding of us is the General Health Questionnaire, or the GHQ. The GHQ does not identify or diagnose specific disorders; rather, it is used as a broad assessment of mental health functioning. It is most often used as a World Health Organization screening tool to assess levels of functioning in multiple domains, such as sleep, attention, concentration, eating, and work. It is highly sensitive and meant to identify individuals within a population that may have, or be at risk to develop, common psychiatric disorders such as depression, anxiety, somatic symptoms, and social withdrawal. It is not specific, nor is it a diagnostic tool (Vieweg & Hedlund, 1983).

The GHQ-30 consists of thirty questions such as "Have you recently been able to enjoy your normal day-to-day activities?" and "Have you recently been finding it easy to get on with other people?" We are asked to choose one of four answers ranging from "not at all" to "much more than usual" based on how we have generally felt over the past few weeks. Using the binary scoring method, the two most symptomatic answers for any given question have a score of "1," while the two least symptomatic answers have a score of "0." Any total sum score of four or above is classified as "psychiatric caseness," which indicates that further attention may be warranted. Scores between five and twenty are common and usually mean that you are going through some important life changes and stressors. Scores between twenty-one and thirty usually should be followed up with an appointment or discussion with your doctor or mental health specialists to see what specifically might be the problem and what needs to be done to fix it (Goldberg, Oldehinkel, & Ormel, 1998).

As one would guess, having a high score on this screen usually makes it harder to do the exercises that we have lined up for you.

Facts About You (FAY)

The Facts About You (FAY) is a demographic and general functioning questionnaire. It is also known as the Meaning of Life (MOL).

Like the GHQ, the FAY does not identify or diagnose specific disorders. Rather, it asks demographic questions, such as gender, sex, ethnicity, age, level of education, occupation, and basic medical history. The results help situate us within the population at large. This information gives an idea of the obstacles and aids we may have in accessing our motivational unconscious, allowing us to tailor an individual approach to this work. For example, females tend to have an easier time accessing their emotions and unconscious than males, as do those with higher levels of education. People from certain cultures, such as Germanic, Nordic European, and some Eastern Asian cultures, like the Japanese—cultures that place a premium on muting emotions—may have a harder time with this task. Health problems, especially chronic illness or long-term hospitalization, can increase the difficulty of this work. Those in psychological treatment tend to find it easier because they are already doing this work in some capacity.

The FAY questionnaire also asks us to rate our overall level of happiness with ourselves, school/work, friends, family, and free time, on a scale of 1 (very unhappy) to 9 (very happy). The population means and standard deviations for these scores are in the following table. Standard deviation (SD) measures dispersity, or how much the scores in a set vary from the average in a population. It describes the distribution of a group of scores. For example, a "happiness with family" mean score of 7.1 with a standard deviation of 2.0 indicates that the population average for happiness with family is 7.1, and 68 percent of people score between 5.1 and 9. A score that falls between the mean and one half of a standard deviation is within the normal range, while one that falls between one half of a standard deviation and one standard deviation is likely to be outside the normal range. A score outside one standard deviation is considered to be outside the normal range.

The graph on the next page is a Gaussian, or bell, curve, which is a visual representation of the normal distribution of scores in a population. Most people score within one standard deviation of the mean, plus or minus. This group of people is depicted by the area under the curve between "–1 SD" and "+1 SD." As the line gets farther away from the mean in either direction, the area under the curve gets smaller, which means fewer people score in that range.

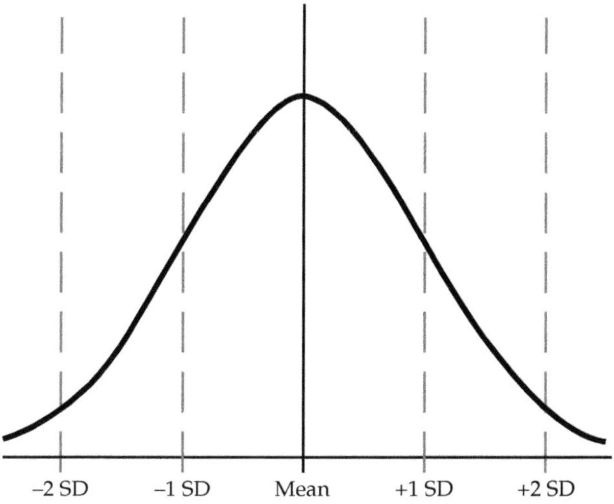

Those who are statistically inclined might want to calculate the z-score, which is a measure of how many standard deviations the score is from the population mean. The formula for calculating a z-score is: z = [(the score)—(population mean)]/(the standard deviation). It can be calculated for all the psychometric measurements discussed here, except for the GHQ.

	Population mean	*Standard deviation*	*1 Standard deviation range*	*½ Standard deviation*	*½ Standard deviation range*
Happiness with Family	7.1	2.0	5.1–9.0	1.0	6.1–8.1
Happiness with Friends	7.4	1.8	5.6–9.0	0.9	6.5–8.3
Happiness with Work	6.2	2.1	4.1–8.3	1.1	5.1–7.3
Happiness with Recreation	7.0	2.0	5.0–9.0	1.0	6.0–8.0
Overall Happiness	7.0	1.8	5.2–8.8	0.9	6.1–7.9

These questions are designed for the subject to self-report functioning within the four general domains of his life: interpersonal, academic/vocational, recreational, and bodily maintenance. They also provide information regarding the balance in our lives. For example, if we heavily prioritize work, we would have high scores in this category, but lower scores in other categories. These scores therefore give a general indication of how well we are functioning in each category.

The Weinberger Adjustment Inventory (WAI-84)

The Weinberger Adjustment Inventory (WAI) is a self-reported questionnaire that assesses overall character traits and adaptive styles (Weinberger & Schwartz, 1990). It also determines personality typologies, which provide information about behavioral tendencies, expected ease of accessing emotions, and potential obstacles in accessing the motivational unconscious (Khanzode, Kraemer, Saxena, Chang, & Steiner, 2006). By virtue of being self-reported, the WAI results reflect who we think we are. This self-construction has proven to be largely accurate and relatively stable over time. While there may be some distortions in how we see ourselves, the WAI has been designed to take these distortions into account and has been proven to be a valid and reliable measure. It is similar to much more extensive assessments, such as the *Minnesota Multiphasic Personality Inventory* (*MMPI*) and the *The Millon Clinical Multiaxial Inventory*, as my and other colleagues' research has shown. It also summarizes four of the traits that have been identified across many decades and theoretical systems as the most important in personality research. We have modified this scale in a series of studies to make it simpler and better suited for use.

The WAI asks us to respond to eighty-four statements about how we have usually felt or acted over the past year or more. The length of this time frame is important, as it asks us to summarize behavior and thoughts over longer periods of time, unlike the GHQ which gives a snapshot of how we feel right now. The WAI questions aim to gauge how we generally think and behave, rather than how we may react to a specific situation. A score significantly higher or lower than the age-matched mean in any of these categories would indicate that we generally experience more or less, respectively, of the given variable than the average person. The standard deviation for all WAI scores is 0.5, meaning that a difference of 0.5 above or below the age-matched mean is considered significant.

Before you delve into the details of this screen, you need to have a quick look at your set score, or validity score. It needs to be a minimum of 3.7. If you score lower than 3.7, the rest of your WAI results will not be accurate. The validity score simply measures whether or not you read the scale accurately and understood some of its double negatives. Many people score a perfect 5.0 on this subscale, which definitely gives you the green light to go ahead and study your results on the other WAI subscales.

The first of these scores is Distress, which is comprised of anxiety, anger, and depression scores. It is a measure of our propensity to access and experience negative emotions. The second score is Positive Emotions, which is comprised of happiness and self-esteem scores. Each of these emotions teaches us something and serves an adaptive purpose, even those that we consider negative. Sadness causes us to withdraw, giving us time to reevaluate. Anxiety and fear increase alertness, caution, and learning. Anger motivates us to stand up for ourselves and our own, to defend ourselves from attack, and to set things straight in response to disappointment.

Our emotions provide the compass that guides us through life, and in order to learn from them, we must allow ourselves to feel them. Therefore, it serves us to have a reasonable amount of access to our emotions, which is indicated by a score within 0.5 of the age-matched mean. A significantly higher score can indicate a level of access that can create an overwhelming flood of emotional information. On the other end of the spectrum, a score significantly below the age-matched mean may indicate a lack of emotionality, which can also be maladaptive, because without emotion, we lose track of what is important to attend to.

The remaining three WAI scores measure conscious and unconscious self-regulation processes. Restraint is a measure of the self-regulation processes that we consciously employ, with some effort, to control our behavior and emotions. The Restraint score is comprised of impulse control, consideration of others, and responsibility scores. By exercising these processes, we control our behavior even though we may feel otherwise inclined. For example, these processes keep us from behaving violently when we feel angry. Being somewhat high in Restraint will facilitate participation in the exercises in this book, to a degree. It gives us some feelings of security and a sense that, as we embark upon this emotional journey of self-discovery, we will not lose our grip on steering the process. We are in command. However, if we are too restrained, we will find it difficult to follow the lead of our emotions, especially our negative ones.

The final two scores, Repressive Defensiveness and Denial of Distress, reflect automatic self-regulation processes that we unconsciously employ when under stress. In Freudian theory, they are called defenses. They prevent us from consciously experiencing a certain amount of distress. In comparison to Restraint, Repressive Defensiveness and Denial of Distress happen automatically and without our conscious awareness or effort. A good example of repressive forgetting was given in Chapter One, when I forgot to attend a talk being given by a physician whom I did not care for. I did not consciously, deliberately, miss the talk; rather my dislike for the speaker unconsciously and automatically motivated me to forget about the talk completely.

While Repressive Defensiveness and Denial of Distress serve a similar purpose, they are distinct processes. Denial of Distress is an unconscious minimization of negative feelings. Someone denying his distress may acknowledge his stressful situation, but the amount of distress he consciously experiences will be disproportionately minimized compared to reality. He may say, "Yeah, I have cancer, but it's not that bad." His unconscious self-regulation process protects him from the full extent of his distress, though he retains some awareness of reality. By permitting him to experience some emotion, Denial of Distress allows for some learning from the event, although his minimization of the importance of the event and his emotions can be problematic. Research has indicated that a certain amount of denial helps to survive immediately stressful, and even life threatening, situations, such as being in the intensive care unit after a heart attack. In the long run, however, continued denial would become increasingly problematic, because it would prevent one from recognizing the lifestyle factors that have led to the heart attack in the first place and from instituting new behaviors, such as quitting smoking, losing weight, and eating a healthy diet.

Repressive Defensiveness, on the other hand, is an automatic process in which we fully repress the experience of distress, thereby eliminating these negative emotions from our consciousness. In some ways, the label "repression," which derives from classic analysis, is probably a misnomer. The actual process by which we "repress," or forget, a problematic event is most likely closer to non-elaboration. By not discussing or thinking about the details of a situation, we lay down only weak memory tracks, which are rapidly erased as other experiences crowd them out. In doing so, we create a discrepancy between our experience and reality. Someone with a fear of the dentist may completely forget to go to a dental appointment. She does not experience distress in relation to the stressor; rather, she eliminates the entire situation from her conscious experience. Repressive Defensiveness strips an event of its emotional content and thus eliminates the possibility of learning from the emotion or experience. As with Denial of Distress, completely repressing the experience and the consequent emotions of having a heart attack also decreases the chances of adopting a healthier lifestyle.

Each of these processes relates somewhat differently to the upcoming exercises. Repressive Defensiveness tends to make them more difficult, while Denial of Distress somewhat facilitates them.

In addition to providing these measures of functioning, the WAI assigns us to one of four personality typologies, each with a distinct profile and set of characteristics. Such a summation into a "type" is very convenient, because instead of keeping all these separate scores and subscales in mind, types contain typical admixtures of each. However, the danger of typing someone is, as always, that not everyone fits a type and not all types are exclusive. Being human makes us complicated.

To arrive at what type you are, plot your Distress and Restraint scores on their respective axes, as depicted in the graph on the next page. This places you within one of the four quadrants, which each represents a personality type: Reactive, Non-Reactive, Suppressor, and Repressor. The X-axis represents Restraint, and the Y-axis represents Distress. The point of intersection is given by the appropriate Distress and Restraint age-matched means.

If one's Distress score is higher than his age-matched mean, and his Restraint score is lower than his age-matched mean, he is classified as Reactive. Lower than average Distress and Restraint scores are characteristic of the Non-Reactive personality. The Suppressor personality is defined by high Distress and high Restraint scores, and the Repressor personality is characterized by low Distress and high Restraint.

Distress and Restraint age-matched means.

	Ages 11–12	*Ages 12–17*	*Ages 17–30*	*Ages 31–60*
Restraint	3.7	3.7	3.6	4.1
Distress	2.7	2.6	2.6	2.2
Point of Intersection between Restraint & Distress	(3.7, 2.7)	(3.7, 2.6)	(3.6, 2.6)	(4.1, 2.2)

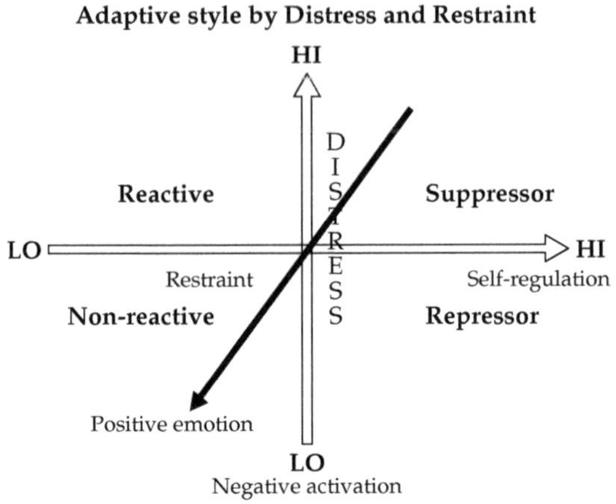

For example, for those between the ages seventeen and thirty, the Restraint line (X-axis) intersects the Distress line (Y-axis) on the above graph at (3.6, 2.6). So, if a twenty-five-year-old man's Restraint score was higher than 3.6, he would fall into the Suppressor or Repressor category. If his Distress score was then higher than 2.6, he would be a Suppressor; if his Distress score was lower than 2.6, he would be a Repressor. On the other hand, if his Restraint score was lower than 3.6, he would fall into the Reactive or Non-Reactive category. In that case, a Distress score that was higher than 2.6 would put him in the Reactive category, while a Distress score lower than 2.6 would put him in the Non-Reactive category.

For those thirty-one years or older, the two lines intersect at (4.1, 2.2) on the above graph. Therefore, a fifty-year-old woman with a Restraint score of 4.2 (i.e., higher than 4.1) would be in the Suppressor or Repressor category. A Distress score of 2.3 (i.e., higher than 2.2) would put her in the Suppressor category, while a Distress score of 2.1 (i.e., lower than 2.2) would put her in the Repressor category. Conversely, if the same woman scored a 3.9 on Restraint (i.e., lower than 4.1), she would be either a Reactive or Non-Reactive personality type. A Distress score above 2.2 would put her in the Reactive category, while a Distress score below 2.2 would put her in the Non-Reactive category.

Each of these personality types is associated with a distinct set of behaviors and characteristics. We adopt these different adaptive styles in order to handle stress, and none is considered intrinsically better or worse than any other. Each type is merely a unique personality flavor with its own particular pros and cons.

Reactive individuals (low Restraint and high Distress) access negative and stressful emotions with ease but do not readily regulate their behavior and emotional reactions. Their lack of conscious regulation leads to a high level of impulsivity, which when combined with high Distress, produces strong emotions that are not well-contained. When faced with a stressor, the Reactive individual would typically feel and display strong emotions. The advantage to such an adaptive style emerges in a dangerous situation, where reacting is important, such as witnessing a fight. Reactive individuals would quickly remove themselves from such a situation. The exercises in this book will likely be very stimulating for them, but might also propel them down a very emotional path.

The Non-Reactive personality (low Distress and low Restraint) is characterized by an overall low level of affect. People who fall into this category do not have easy access to emotions. They are often quite stoic. To others, they may seem lackadaisical. This personality type also has low levels of conscious self-regulation, indicating greater than usual impulsivity, diminished consideration for others, and a reduced sense of responsibility. This combination can create less need for social approval. They are sometimes hard to motivate to do things that they find difficult and that require effort on their part. Non-Reactive individuals are not easily affected by stressful situations, and they may feel confused by the emotional reactions that, for example, a Reactive individual may display. Such individuals would probably succeed in exciting and even dangerous environments where the ability to persevere rather than react is advantageous, such as in combat or on Wall Street. The exercises in this book will challenge Non-Reactive people; they may find them irrelevant, or even boring.

The Suppressor, characterized by high Distress and high Restraint, can both access and consciously contain strong emotions. These individuals do not negate their emotions, but high levels of self-regulation allow them to control when and how they express them. Thus, they can access emotions when appropriate and put them aside when needed. Their high level of self-regulation also results in lower impulsivity. Suppressive people likely have an advantage when acting or writing creatively; both activities call for easy access to, and the ability to control, emotions of all kinds. They also might find it easy to be empathetic listeners or to be in psychotherapy themselves. In my experience, students with this profile tend to find the exercises in this book relatively easy, as many of them have already tried these kinds of exercises on their own. In psychotherapy, such individuals usually benefit quickly and improve rapidly. They make my job as a clinician easier than most of the other types.

Finally, the Repressor is defined by low Distress and high Restraint. Like Suppressors, Repressors show low impulsivity, but unlike Suppressors they have difficulty accessing their emotions and do not easily acknowledge the presence of negative emotions, to themselves or others. In contrast to Non-Reactives, who show low levels of affect, Repressors exert such a high degree of regulation over their emotions that their feelings are buried away. They may show unconscious signs of distress, but report no conscious experience of these emotions. Repressors are very tightly controlled people. They do well when things go well, but not when things go badly, especially when circumstances make them appear in an unfavorable light. The exercises in this book will likely go well for Repressors when we inquire about positives, but they may become more difficult when we ask them to report on more stressful events.

There is a linear relationship between the Distress and Restraint scores and the degree to which these behaviors and personality tendencies are exhibited. The farther away (higher or lower) the Distress and/or the Restraint scores are from the age-matched mean, the more extreme the associated behaviors become. Depending on circumstances, our scores can migrate toward or away from the age-matched mean, but they typically remain within a particular quadrant. Stress can significantly affect where we fall on this spectrum at any given time, moving us toward the extreme of our personality type. For example, when faced with a stressor a Reactive individual is likely to become more distressed and less restrained. A Repressor, on the other hand, is likely to become more self-regulated. In short, we become caricatures of ourselves when we operate in a difficult psychosocial context. By bringing us closer to the age-matched mean, therapy and other self-discovery tools can ameliorate maladaptive behaviors sometimes associated with the extreme versions of each personality type.

Age and gender also affect these scores. Women tend to score higher on Distress and are more likely than men to be Reactives or Suppressors. Men, on the other hand, tend to score lower on Distress and are more often Non-Reactives and Repressors. Because over time we tend to become more self-regulated, Restraint scores increase with age. While our scores might alter significantly within a category due to age and stress, our personality type usually does not change.

Understanding our own personality type and tendencies can provide valuable information about the ease or difficulty we may encounter when we try to access our own motivational unconscious. While some personality types may present unique obstacles to accessing the unconscious, none is insurmountable. Reactive types typically have the ability to access their emotions, but have difficulty controlling them. Delving into the unconscious can unearth significant emotion, which may be overwhelming. Non-Reactive individuals can find this task difficult due to their lower level of emotional awareness and understanding. Difficulty in accessing emotions can, in turn, create challenges to accessing the unconscious, and potentially create a lack of motivation to do so. For those in the Repressor category, a high level of self-regulation can be a challenging obstacle to accessing their emotions, which have often been repressed into their unconscious. On the other hand, that same high level of self-control can serve to motivate them to work diligently at the task. Of the four personality types, Suppressors are likely to have the easiest time unlocking and analyzing their unconscious. Their baseline level of emotional awareness eases the task, and their ability to exert control over their emotions means they may find the process less overwhelming than the Reactives do.

We are all capable of understanding our own unconscious processes more deeply, regardless of the obstacles our specific personality tendencies may present. Understanding these tendencies actually helps us to overcome these obstacles. In this regard, knowledge is power.

The WAI and the Big Five Personality model by McCrae and Costa

We have discussed how the WAI is a quick and easy measure of personality. For those of you interested in learning more, let us discuss briefly what we and other researchers have found about the Big Five Personality model by Robert McCrae and Paul Costa (2008). The five-factor model of personality consists of five broad domains of personality: Openness to Experience, Conscientiousness, Extraversion, Agreeableness, and Neuroticism. Openness to Experience assesses the degree to which we are intellectually curious, adventurous, appreciative of art, creative, and independent. Conscientiousness measures self-discipline, planned vs. spontaneous behavior, dependability, and organization. A high score in

Conscientiousness indicates a tendency to strive for high achievement. Extraversion refers to our sociability and talkativeness. It also measures positive emotions, energy, and assertiveness. Agreeableness evaluates our tendency to be cooperative, compassionate, trusting, and helpful. Finally, Neuroticism is a measure of our negative emotions, such as anger, anxiety, and depression.

Scores on the Big Five Personality Test are reported as percentiles. An 80 percent score for Extraversion means that 80 percent of people who have taken the test are less extraverted and 20 percent are more so. Scores within the 40th to 60th percentile are considered average. These results are not as specific as psychometrics like the WAI, but they do give a general idea of personality tendencies.

The Big Five Personality Test measures similar personality dimensions as the WAI. As shown in the table below, the WAI variable Restraint measures characteristics similar to both Conscientiousness and Agreeableness, Extraversion is similar to Positive Emotions, and Neuroticism is fairly equivalent to Distress. However, there is no WAI equivalent variable for Openness to Experience or for Agreeableness, and the Big Five does not measure Repressive Defensiveness or Denial of Distress.

While these correlations are not exact and the Big Five does not break down each variable into subscales, it is a good alternative that will give similar feedback when the WAI is not accessible. One of the major advantages of using the Big Five Personality Test is that it is easily accessible and affordable. The test can be found online free of charge. For more information about how the Big Five correlates with the WAI, please refer to Daniel Weinberger's publications.

Comparison of WAI and Big 5 Personality Test Variables.

WAI	*Big 5*
No equivalent	Openness to Experience
Restraint	Conscientiousness
Positive emotions	Extraversion
Restraint	Agreeableness
Distress	Neuroticism
Repressive Defensiveness	No equivalent
Denial of Distress	No equivalent

The heart rate exercise

Now, let's do a simple heart rate exercise, which will give you further information about your degree of emotional access and restraint. After at least five minutes of rest, count your resting heart rate by placing your index and middle fingers of one hand on the inside wrist of your other arm. Alternatively, place your index and middle fingers of one hand on your neck, just under your jaw line, slightly to the right. When you feel your pulse, count the beats for a full minute and take note. This number reflects your baseline emotional activation, which corresponds to the Distress variable on the WAI below.

Then, stand up and immediately count your pulse for another full minute. This is your challenge heart rate, which reflects your ability to regulate your emotions. This number corresponds to the Restraint variable on the WAI below.

For most people, their heart rate increases slightly when they stand up. The average resting heart rate is 76 (with a standard deviation of 10), and the average challenge heart rate is 86 (with a standard deviation of 10). Variables such as your height, weight, BMI (average = 22; standard deviation = 2.3; BMI calculator: http://www.cdc.gov/healthyweight/assessing/bmi/adult_bmi/english_bmi_calculator/bmi_calculator.html), caffeine consumption, medications, illness, and nutrition, among others, can impact your resting and challenge heart rate.

However, in general, if your resting and/or challenge heart rate differs from the average by more than 0.5 standard deviation, this is significant. If your resting heart rate is significantly lower than average, that indicates a lower than average level of emotionality; a higher than average resting heart rate indicates a high level of emotionality. A lower than average challenge heart rate indicates a low level of restraint; a high challenge heart rate indicates a high level of restraint. Please refer back to the section on the WAI for a more in-depth discussion of emotionality and restraint.

The Response Evaluation Measure (REM-71)

The last test we ask you to complete takes you squarely into the center of psychodynamic psychology. The Response Evaluation Measure (REM-71) is a self-reported questionnaire that measures classical Freudian defenses. Defenses are highly reflexive, automatic reactions meant to protect us from the awareness of stressors and negative emotions. They also help us to maintain our ability to act quickly in the face of adversity, while preserving our sense of identity and self. In doing so, they can obscure our perception of reality.

Here is an example of how defenses affect our behavior and perception of reality: When I was starting out in my life as a psychiatrist, hours were long and money was tight. I was working two jobs just to make ends meet. On one particular payday, I was at work, quietly finishing up my reports. While I did so, the woman who handled payroll—let's call her Xanthippe—walked in and began banging around the room, looking for something as loudly as possible. Xanthippe was not a very kind or considerate woman. I was tired, under pressure, and irritable, and I grew increasingly angry with her inconsiderate interruption of my work. However, I knew she was revengeful, and I was aware of the less than stellar chances of my paycheck arriving on time should I have expressed my irritation. Finally Xanthippe left, slamming the door behind her. Just then, as I sat there seething, the Coca-Cola man arrived to fill the Coke machine in the hallway, and he was noisy. I leapt out of my chair, stormed out, and yelled "What the hell are you doing?!" The poor Coca-Cola man looked stunned. He was just doing his job and certainly did not deserve this outburst. I, however, felt much better and went back into the office to finish up my reports. I got my work done, received my paycheck on time, and got rid of my anger. The price I paid was losing the Coca Cola man's esteem and making a fool out of myself, but since this was a rare encounter, and I only drink Pepsi anyway, the cost was not too great.

This example demonstrates an automatic defense process called displacement. It occurred within split seconds, and I neither planned nor thought when I yelled at the Coke man; I just reflexively acted. We kick the dog or, in this case, yell at the Coke man, when we are mad at the boss, in order to release an emotion without the consequences. All of us do things like this, and we can benefit from being aware of the defenses that we ourselves tend to employ and how they affect our behavior.

Defenses are natural processes that we all use; they are not intrinsically indicative of pathology. However, some defenses lead to more adaptive functioning, while some are less adaptive. We all favor these processes to varying degrees. The REM measures to what degree we employ the twenty-one different defenses. We are asked to rate seventy-one statements, such as "I go out of my way to help people," and "I laugh at myself pretty easily," on a scale of 1 (disagree) to 9 (agree). The REM gives scores for each of the twenty-one defenses. The standard deviation for all scores is 0.5. Scores that are 0.5 or more above or below the age-matched mean are considered significant.

The twenty-one defenses measured by the REM are separated into two categories: Factor 1 includes fourteen defenses, and Factor 2 includes the remaining seven. Each factor is then subdivided into Interpersonal Defenses, which are processes that influence behavioral dynamics with others, and Intrapsychic Defenses, which are internal mental processes that influence our thoughts and perceptions. The REM provides the total Factor 1 and Factor 2 scores.

The Factor 1 score is a measure of the tendency to assimilate reality to fit within preexisting beliefs and perceptions. When we employ Factor 1 defenses, we do not adjust ourselves according to experience; instead, we adjust our perception of reality according to our existing internal landscape and what we already believe to be true. For example, in a conflict, Factor 1 defenses cause us to blame others rather than to think about how we might handle the situation differently next time. A Factor 1 defense is considered the less mature defense mechanism, as it does not allow for learning and growth. Factor 1 correlates moderately with Repressive Defensiveness on the WAI.

The Factor 2 score, or accommodation, measures the tendency to absorb external information and make some relevant internal adjustments. If we score high in Factor 2, we tend to somewhat change ourselves to comply with what we learn about reality, rather than changing reality to fit within what we already believe. To a certain degree, these defenses are more likely to cause us to adjust our own behavior rather than entirely blame another person in a conflict. Factor 2 defenses also facilitate positive reactions, such as humor, during stressful experiences. Factor 2 defenses correlate moderately with Denial of Distress on the WAI, and they are considered more helpful and more mature mechanisms than Factor 1 defenses.

The 21 defenses are classified and defined as follows:

Factor 1 Interpersonal Defenses

Acting out

The process of using actions rather than feelings or reflections to deal with a stressor.

- Sample Item: When I am upset I do things without thinking.

Displacement

The transference of a feeling from one object or person to another, usually less threatening, object or person. For example, an employee who is angry with his boss may turn around and direct these feelings toward a subordinate employee. The motivation behind displacement is to allow for a less consequential emotional release by targeting a less threatening person or object.

- Sample Item: I won't let people in authority know I'm angry at them, but everyone else better watch out!

Passive-aggression

Dealing with a stressor by indirectly expressing negative feelings towards other people.

- Sample Item: If someone is unfair to me I probably won't do what I told them I'd do.

Projection

An individual deals with a stressor by incorrectly attributing her own feelings or thoughts to other people. For example, Projection would cause an individual who feels angry to perceive anger in others, instead of acknowledging her own emotion.

- Sample Item: I am usually treated unfairly.

Splitting

An individual compartmentalizes positive and negative qualities of himself or others, rather than integrating both into a cohesive image. Splitting prevents an individual from seeing shades of grey between good and bad, particularly in interpersonal relationships.

- Sample Item: When someone I like lets me down, I usually trust them again.

Withdrawal

The process of removing oneself from social interactions or from experiencing reality.

- Sample Item: When things upset me I'd rather be by myself.

Factor 1 Intrapsychic Defenses

Conversion

An individual experiences physical symptoms, such as paralysis or breathing difficulties, which have no physiological cause and have a very odd anatomical distribution that conflicts with our knowledge of how nerves work. Very often the reported symptom can be read by the observer (but not by the reporter) as a symbol of the underlying stressor. For example, an individual may have a paralyzed hand after wanting to strike his elderly parent.

- Sample Item: Sometimes I have lost all the feeling in one part of my body and nobody could explain why.

Dissociation

A process of detaching from reality by temporarily changing one's character or sense of personal identity. This defense can involve a breakdown in the functioning of various processes, such as consciousness, memory, self-perception, perception of the environment, and motor/ sensory behavior.

- Sample Item: I often get the feeling that whatever is going on is not really happening to me.

Fantasy

An individual handles stress through excessive daydreaming rather than problem solving the situation. Daydreaming can also replace interpersonal relationships.

- Sample Item: I like to imagine that my life is very different.

Omnipotence

An individual deals with stressors by feeling or acting superior to others, including feeling or acting as if she has special powers or abilities.

- Sample Item: I don't want to brag, but usually I'm the one who knows how to get things done.

Repression

An individual copes with distressing thoughts or experiences by eliminating these stressors from her conscious awareness.

- Sample Item: When I should have strong feelings, I don't feel anything.

Somatization

An individual expresses psychological distress in the form of physical symptoms, without symbolic content. His complaint does not "stand for" anything; he simply reports illness and pain. His distress could be due to existing pain that provides a focus and a model, but his report is out of line with the magnitude of the cause of pain. For example, a stress headache might lead to hours in bed. His distress may also relate to worries about pain that signals a dire event, such as a recurrence of cancer.

- Sample Item: When I get stressed I get ill really easily.

Sublimation

The process of channeling maladaptive thoughts or feelings into behavior that is socially acceptable.

- Sample Item: I like to write stories or poems when I've just been through a really rough situation.

Undoing

An individual uses words or behaviors to symbolically make amends for unacceptable thoughts or behaviors or to minimize them.

- Sample Item: I repeat special thoughts or words over and over to myself when I am uptight or frightened.

Factor 2 Interpersonal Defenses

Altruism

An individual handles stressors by working to help or support others, which gives him a vicarious sense of gratification.

- Sample Item: I go out of my way to help people.

Humor

An individual focuses on the amusing aspects of the stressor, and she uses comedy to express and release otherwise distressing feelings or thoughts.

- Sample Item: When things go wrong, I can still see the funny side.

Idealization

The individual attributes excessive positive qualities to others. Consequently, he perceives other people as "good" or "bad" people, with no grey area. The mechanism leads him to reject the good or bad in himself.

- Sample Item: I know this great person whose advice I can usually trust.

Reaction formation

The individual substitutes an unacceptable thought, feeling, or impulse for its opposite.

- Sample Item: Often I act really nice when actually I am pretty upset.

Factor 2 Intrapsychic Defenses

Denial (isolation of affect)

The individual avoids emotional distress by separating an idea from its associated feelings.

- Sample Item: When I am upset I remind myself that everything is really okay.

Intellectualization

An individual excessively uses abstract thinking to avoid or minimize disturbing emotions.

- Sample Item: I use reason and logic, not feelings, to understand people.

Suppression

An individual consciously avoids thinking about distressing thoughts or emotions.

- Sample Item: When I need to, I can put my problems on hold until later when I can think about them.

Each of us habitually favors and employs different defense mechanisms to varying degrees. These tendencies are reinforced when we are young; different childhood experiences and environments produce different defense mechanism portfolios. As we go through life, our socialization determines the extent to which we overcome or alter any of our maladaptive defense mechanisms. Growing up under adverse circumstances often makes it more difficult to overcome defenses learned at an early age. Additionally, trauma tends to produce a particular defense profile of high scores in Projection, Splitting, Conversion, Dissociation, and Repression. Age affects these scores; young people tend to score higher in Factor 1 than Factor 2, a pattern that reflects a lack of maturity and life experience.

The degree to which we employ different defenses provides information about how easy or difficult it may be to access the motivational unconscious. Generally, those who score high in Factor 1 and low in Factor 2 find the techniques used to access the unconscious, such as expressive writing and dream analysis, difficult, but high scorers on either Factor 1 or Factor 2 can find the exercises challenging. Knowing which defenses we favor informs us about our own potential obstacles to accessing the unconscious and thus gives us clues about how to overcome these obstacles.

Understanding our own defense mechanisms helps us see how we unconsciously view and interact with the world. As some defense mechanisms are more adaptive than others, it is helpful to recognize the maladaptive defense mechanisms that are not serving us. If we score particularly high or low on a defense parameter compared to the norm for our age, we might need help. Because different defenses are appropriate for different circumstances, it is helpful to maintain a broad portfolio of these processes, rather than a single defense mechanism for all stressors. Gaining information about our own tendencies and defense styles gives us the opportunity to develop more adaptive thoughts and behaviors. Though these processes are unconscious, a certain amount of self-knowledge and awareness can give us some control.

CHAPTER FOUR

An easy start: memes, slips of the tongue and ear, and parapraxes

Memes

I now begin a series of chapters that discuss different exercises designed to help you access and understand your motivational unconscious. These exercises may not immediately flow quickly and freely for all; some personality traits may make this journey difficult. In the previous chapter I highlighted some of these traits, such as Repressive Defensiveness and, to some extent, Denial of Distress. To prepare for your own potential obstacles, take another look at your scores from the psychometrics we discussed previously. Stress, too, may increase your difficulty with these tasks. When we are very stressed it becomes difficult to contemplate complex issues; where there is crisis, there is no analysis.

Even if all your traits are in line with exploration, there is still a need for practice: For most there is a learning curve that requires reading a variety of examples in addition to practicing the exercises. For each task I will provide samples extracted from my own personal experience, famous cases, or my past students. I couple these practical exercises and examples with a discussion of the current theory and the supporting empirical evidence for each technique in order to show you how these exercises can aid in your own process of self-discovery.

First, let's discuss how taking a look at our personal memes, or the rules that we live by, can give us valuable insight into our unconscious belief systems, motivations, and behavioral patterns. The British evolutionary biologist, Richard Dawkins, first introduced the term "meme" in 1976. It refers to a unit of cultural information that is transmitted verbally or by repeated action from one mind to another. Most are familiar with internet memes, which are concepts—pictures and quotes, for example—that spread from person to person via the internet. These are a subset of the kind of meme we will work with here.

Memes were intended to be the cultural analogy to genes, which are the biological units of inheritance. While genes determine how the biological characteristics of a species persist, disappear, or change over time, memes serve a similar cultural purpose; they are the units of cultural evolution. Just as genetic inheritance might cause us to have the same hair color as our parents, the intergenerational transmission of memes between people lead us to the same beliefs and attitudes as our parents (McNamara, 2011).

In order to bring up the memes that you live by, it is usually easiest to remember the kind of dinner conversations you had in your family, or the kind of "parental talks" and admonishments you received as a child, especially when you transgressed or made some big personal decisions in education, work, or partner choice. While memes are easily brought into our consciousness through deliberate analysis, most of the time they reside in our unconscious. We are normally unaware of how these rules influence the way that we live. Memes set automatic and unconscious cultural boundaries for determining what is important in our day-to-day activities. For example, if we grew up with the family meme that vacation is an important aspect of a happy life, we would be unlikely to debate whether or not to go on vacation; we would just plan for an annual vacation. Memes allow us to go on autopilot. Because these unconscious rules influence conscious behaviors and thoughts, they can be thought of as a bridge between the unconscious and the conscious mind. By bringing these unconscious thoughts and beliefs into our awareness, we can begin to understand why we behave the way that we do, and we can make changes to improve how we function and our well-being.

Memes can take on a variety of forms: thoughts, ideas, theories, practices, habits, songs, dances, images, gestures, phrases, and moods, depending on the level of abstraction. As I discussed in

Chapter Two, different spheres of abstraction, from culture to genes, can be used to understand our psychological functioning (please see the "Levels of Abstraction" graphic in Chapter Two). On a larger scale, memes can drive the transmission of culture, languages, religion, ideologies, and political systems. On an individual, personal level, memes can be thought of as the rules that we live by.

At all levels of abstraction, memes replicate via imitation and social learning, as defined by Albert Bandura's work here at Stanford (1997). A symbol becomes a meme rather than an abstract stimulus when we have learned what the symbol means and how to communicate that concept to another person. Memes are not innate, they are not hardwired within us; rather, they are learned through observation. In 1982 the Italian geneticist Luigi Luca Cavalli-Sforza and his colleagues demonstrated this point with research that showed that the transmission of political ideals is primarily familial, rather than genetic. In other words, they verified that we do not acquire our political beliefs genetically, but through observation and imitation.

But memes are not always easily accepted and integrated, especially if they put us in conflict with what is common belief of the time. Children sometimes know the familial memes, but reject them. This finding is no surprise: Many children have different political orientations from their parents. In fact, very often children will adopt conflicting political views as a form of protest and rebellion. Another example may be the change in attitudes regarding sexual orientation that has taken place in the past ten years.

Memes must be learned, and we learn our memes as children from those who surround us. We internalize the memes of our families or caregivers. Living as closely and dependently as we do with our families of origin, for as long as we do, we absorb these rules through social modeling and learning. Oftentimes, these rules that we pick up from our parents persist into adulthood and continue to influence who we are and how we behave. By examining the rules and sayings we grew up with, we begin to understand what rules we unconsciously live by.

Animal studies have begun to unearth the potential neural basis of the transmission of memes from one person to another. In studies with monkeys, neurons called mirror neurons have been found to be involved in recognizing the intention of others and in imitation. When a monkey saw the experimenter grasp food in a certain way, the specific motor neurons that fired in the monkey's brain were the same ones that fired when the monkey itself grasped the food. The monkey's brain mirrored the observed action. These same mirror neurons have been hypothesized to be responsible for the evolution of language and empathy and for the replication of memes in humans. However, the neuronal mechanisms of these processes are likely to be quite complex. Confirming these findings will require a great deal more scientific inquiry.

One important difference between genes and memes is that while both replicate over generations, genetic evolution occurs gradually, over long periods of time. Memes, on the other hand, can be reconstructed and reshaped within a single generation. They are interesting from the point of view of adaptation, because we can change and eliminate our own maladaptive memes. Our lives are not necessarily at the mercy of all the beliefs and ideas that our families and cultures have passed along to us. Instead, by undertaking an honest analysis and introspection of our own unconscious rules, we can create healthier and more adaptive memes. We can become better suited to live in the environments we have sought out and, to some extent, created for ourselves.

To find your own memes, think about the words of wisdom or life lessons your parents or caregivers told you. Throughout your childhood, you probably heard repeated phrases or sayings. Imagine your parents coming home from work, or being with you in a pleasant vacation setting, expounding the values of life. What did they used to tell you? The example below is a list of phrases I used to hear my father say as he took off his shoes and got ready for a relaxed dinner at home:

- "Work [sport, vacation, or whatever the activity at hand was] is the most beautiful thing"
- "You have to eat heartily to be healthy"
- "Behave: you are a guest of nature"
- "When there is a need the devil eats flies"
- "The situation is hopeless but not serious".

These five memes have had a significant impact on my values, perspective, and lifestyle. As emphasized in meme #1, "Work [sport, vacation] is the most beautiful thing," maintaining balance among work, athletics, and leisure has always been important to me. While I am devoted to my career, I always take advantage of every minute of vacation and sabbatical time available, in contrast to many of my colleagues. One in particular used to stay in the lab until 10 pm every night—sometimes even sleeping there—with no weekends, vacations, sabbaticals, or holidays. I, on the other hand, preferred to be home by 6 pm almost every day in order to have dinner with my family, and I have never turned down a vacation opportunity.

In line with meme #2, I believe that eating well and enjoying culinary delights are important aspects of well-being, and I have even devoted a significant portion of my professional efforts to helping individuals with eating disorders. Meme #3, "Behave: you are a guest of nature," a particularly Austrian attitude, has significantly influenced my lifestyle. I tend to spend vacations in the outdoors, and my respect for nature motivated me to build an eco-friendly house and live a green lifestyle. However, like most others, I am not wedded to my memes: I do drive a Porsche.

Meme #4, "When there is a need, the devil eats flies," reflects the pragmatism and resourcefulness that my family taught me. As much as I appreciate luxury items and fine dining, at the end of the day I make do with what I have. When I was first hired at Stanford, I arrived at the hospital a day early to check things out. I asked the secretary where my office was located, and she unapologetically told me that I did not have one. This was troublesome, as I was scheduled to see patients the next day and now had nowhere to do so. I found a janitor's broom closet, cleaned it out, furnished it with some items straight from my moving truck, and, *voilà*, I had an office.

The final meme, "The situation is hopeless but not serious," reflects the pessimistic, yet lighthearted, attitude toward life that I picked up from my family. Again, this perspective is characteristically Austrian. There is an old joke along these lines, in which a German general and an Austrian general are standing on a hill watching a battle below—a dismal scene. With men dying by the dozen, it begins to rain. The German general clicks his heels, stands up straight, turns to the Austrian general, and says, "Comrade, the situation is serious, but not hopeless." The Austrian general smiles, and says, "Quite the contrary, my friend, the situation is hopeless, but not serious." In my own life, I have adopted this attitude—we do not have the world under our full control, but we can control whether or not we react to it with humor and lightheartedness. These sayings, so casually imparted throughout my childhood, have greatly influenced the way I live my life.

These five sayings are not necessarily congruent, logically aligned, or well thought out. Family memes often openly contradict each other, leaving us to pick and choose which rules to adopt in our own lives. My father might come home one night to say, "Work is the most beautiful thing," and the next evening proclaim, "Vacation is the most beautiful thing." While these contradictions gave me pause as a child, they also gave me the opportunity to select and adapt the memes I wanted to adopt as my own. I could choose to live by the rule that work is the most important thing, vacation is the most important thing, or that a balance between the two is the most important thing.

Memes can be culturally tinged and time stamped: Mine are Austrian memes of the post-World War II period. A recent survey of what Austrians value found their top three choices to be: 1. nature and its protection, 2. time for recreation and play, and 3. good food and drink. My family's own personal set of rules are very much in line with these cultural values. My father expanded them by adding the last two rules, "When there is a need, the devil eats flies," and "The situation is hopeless, but not serious," no doubt reflecting his dismal experiences during World War I, the Austrian Civil War, the Great Depression, and World War II.

Memes from an American family, on the other hand, might be very different. Common American memes include: "God helps those who help themselves," "Stay thin," and "Education is the key to your future." These memes would produce a pattern of behavior and approach to life very different from mine. Living by the rule "You have to eat heartily to be healthy," for example, would create significantly different eating behavior from a rule that staying thin—not food—is the priority in life.

Some excellent books on this subject, in which the authors strive to define different cultures and their significant characteristics, include Luigi Barzini's *The Italians* (1996) and *The Europeans* (1983); Steven Ozment's *A Mighty Fortress* (2004); William M. Johnston's *The Austrian Mind* (1972); Boye Lafayette De Mente's *Kata: The Key to Understanding and Dealing with the Japanese!* (2003); and Robert Frank's book of photographs, *The Americans* (1969).

We must be careful about making assumptions based on country of residence. In America, we are a country of immigrants with different blends of cultural values and expectations. This is also true within families. When two people with different backgrounds marry, two different ways of thinking are imported and blended. Each spouse comes to the table with a different set of memes, and the couple must work to determine the priorities, values, and expectations of the new family.

If you find yourself struggling to identify your own memes, expand your methods. Chat with your parents over a nice meal about what important truths they tried to pass on to you. Ask your siblings what they thought was important when they were growing up in your family. Keep in mind, though, that complete agreement among siblings is the exception rather than the rule. Due to birth order, siblings grow up in both shared and non-shared environments. Although you all grew up in the same family, you did not grow up in exactly the same environment, or with the exact same set of experiences or relationships with each family member. As a result, your siblings may have adopted sets of rules different from yours.

Another way to identify your memes is to let your own children inform you. When you identify what rules you are passing along to your children, you will likely understand what rules were passed along to you. One strategy is to play a role reversal game with your children. Let them be your parent and you the child, and pose common conflicts and problems. You just might be surprised by what they tell you about your memes as they handle your transgressions as a mock child.

Not all of us will adopt our parents' memes as our own. If a rule in the family is hurtful, draconian, or even injurious, most children will reject it and strive to achieve the opposite attitude. A classic example would be the meme, "Spare the rod, spoil the child," in a family where strict discipline derailed into abuse. Abused children often reject this rule. Their own parenting style may become permissive to the extreme. Sometimes, of course, children embrace the injurious prescriptions of the previous generation, thus continuing what Cathy Spatz Widom (1989) has called "the cycle of violence." The ensuing transgenerational transmission of problems perpetuates the ill effects of abuse.

After you have generated your list of memes (usually five to ten of them will stand out), we begin the hermeneutic process of analysis, a method of interpretation similar to the way we might read and interpret the themes in a literary work. Instead of a book or poem, we analyze and seek the deeper meaning of our own behavior and thoughts or, in this case, our family memes. The principle of this hermeneutic process is that we select rules to live by that are meaningful, consciously or unconsciously, from a plethora of inputs.

Memes can be selected because they were uniquely time-stamped and personally important based on experience. Since I grew up amid the economic difficulties of post-World War II Austria, one of my memes is focused on having enough to eat. Sometimes memes are adopted not because they are verbally repeated, but because their sentiment is modeled on a daily basis. My family went for a walk in the woods every single weekend, rain or shine. This act emphasized the importance of nature, and that attitude became a meme of my own. Finally, a meme can be internalized through conscious, willful selection. In other words, when we encounter an attitude or a value that we admire and agree with, we might choose to adopt it as a rule for ourselves. For example, I have adopted my wife's meme that stresses the importance of diversity.

The goal of this exercise is to bring as many of these memes and their significance into our mental work space as possible, so that in the end we can make conscious, informed choices about which ones are precious, which ones to preserve, which ones we will tolerate, which ones we will discard, and which ones we will actively fight to overcome.

First, we ask questions about each of our memes to unearth their deeper meaning. Do you agree with the statement? How does the statement make you feel? Do you have a strong emotional reaction to the statement, either positive or negative? If so, that meme is likely to play an unconscious role in the way you live your life. These steps are the key to the hermeneutic process—you follow your emotional leads, rather than your rational thoughts and beliefs, in order to uncover the personally meaningful connections.

Next, we expand the context of the meme and try to identify its origin. Is it something that your parents often said? Would your parents agree with you? Was the sentiment behind the statement really followed in your family? Or was the opposite often done? Do you remember when those times occurred? How did you react? Consider the historical and cultural context of the meme. Just as my family's memes reflect the culture of post-World War II Austria, your memes may contain a strong infusion of your culture, or the one in which your parents grew up.

Now, think about your current family. If you have children, would they recognize this meme as something they have often heard from you? Would they say that your beliefs and behavior are congruent? Perhaps the most important aspect of this exercise is determining which of your unconscious rules are beneficial and which ones hinder well-being. Ask yourself if you would want to pass this rule along to your children. If you were a child, would this rule energize you, motivate you, and direct you toward positive endeavors, or would it create anxiety, get you into trouble, and become a hindrance in your relationships?

Do you and your partner agree that this is a beneficial meme to live by? If not, how do you think it is negatively affecting you? What would you change?

Finally, what is *not* there is often equally as important as what *is* there. What elements are missing from your set of memes? Do they all more or less refer to the same aspect of life, or are they varied, covering each of the five primary domains of functioning: work/achievement/academics, interpersonal relationships, physical health and fitness, recreation, and psychology and personal reflection?

5 Developmental domains of functioning

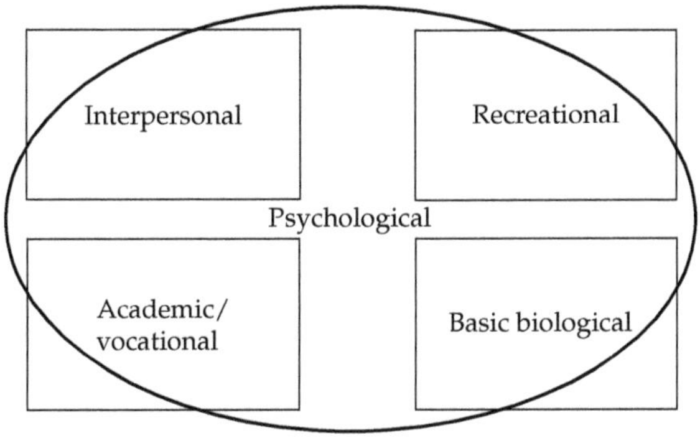

If one—or more—of these aspects of life is missing from your set of memes, why did you omit it? Did your family not emphasize that domain of functioning and not provide a corresponding meme to live by? Have you forgotten the meme from this category? Or did you not like the meme and reject it? What we remember is not necessarily true, and just because we do not remember a meme does not mean that it did not exist. Understanding why certain memes are missing gives us valuable clues about why we live the way we do.

When summarizing all your thoughts about a set of memes, ask yourself if you would like to live in this kind of family, if you had to do it all over again.

One word of caution with this exercise: If you encounter great difficulty finding or discussing any of these memes, even after considerable prompting; if most of the questions above seem irrelevant to you, annoying, or even so intrusive that you simply want to move on; or if, by contrast, your list is endless, extremely contradictory, makes you upset or angry, and stirs up emotional upheaval which you find hard to contain, you might need more than a book can offer. You might need a partner by your side, a guide, or even a professional to help you navigate this journey.

To illustrate how I usually handle this exercise, I will review some memes that previous students brought to class. Because they were of many different nationalities, some of these examples came from students who speak English as a second language. I have taken care not to edit the phrasing of these examples so their meaning is not distorted.

Student 1:

- Try to say "yes" to everything
- You can only regret things you haven't done
- Always have frozen soup in the freezer in case someone is sick and needs it
- Less really *is* more
- Never go to someone's house empty-handed.

What do these memes say? The first, "Try to say 'yes' to everything," is her prescription for interacting with others. According to this rule, she should try to accommodate whatever someone asks of her. The second, "You can only regret things you haven't done," refers to the academic/vocational/achievement domain of functioning: In order to go far in life, she should take every opportunity and participate in every possible experience. Again, the third and fifth statements, "Always have frozen soup in the freezer in case someone is sick and needs it," and "Never go to someone's house empty-handed," refer to her role within interpersonal relationships. The message is that she should always be prepared and willing to take care of others. According to these rules, particularly the last one, manners and politeness are of the utmost importance. "Always have frozen soup in the freezer in case someone is sick and needs it" also addresses physical health by providing a guideline for what to do in the event of illness; however, the meme guides her to take care of others rather than herself. The fourth meme, "Less really *is* more," prescribes a minimalist attitude toward life. This rule is an overarching life philosophy about what is important. It therefore fits within the psychological domain of functioning.

What is missing from this set of rules? Are all five domains of functioning addressed? The main message these memes give is how to satisfy others, but they say very little about how to achieve personal happiness, how to spend free time, or how to keep physically fit. They include no mention of work ethic or education. A child who conforms to this set of rules might grow into an adult who is very focused on other people, and who views herself only in relation to others.

Would you like to live by this set of rules? Do you find these to be positive, helpful memes, or do you think they might promote maladaptive behavior? While the overall message of seizing opportunities and caring for others is arguably a positive teaching, some elements of these memes could produce problematic behavior. Sometimes saying no is okay. Developing the ability to say no comfortably is important, and knowing when to do so is equally important. A focus entirely on pleasing others rather than caring for oneself can also be harmful.

If Student 1 finds herself overwhelmed by over-commitment, unable to say no even when saying yes is not in her best interest, or neglecting her own self-care in favor of caring for others, it would be valuable for her to take a close look at her memes and reevaluate the rules she unconsciously lives by. She can determine which ones to discard, which to tweak, which to keep, and what memes to add to her repertoire.

Student 2:

- Emotional pain is always bearable; physical sometimes isn't
- Take care of yourself when you're going through something
- Live every day as if it's your last.

These memes are a very limited set of rules. Each refers to physical pain or illness to some degree: the first says that sometimes we cannot endure physical pain but we can always tolerate emotional pain; the second affirms the importance of self-care when things are difficult—and we can infer from Student 2's first meme that she is referring to something physically painful; and the third refers to the fragility and uncertainty of life: We should live fully today, because—who knows—death may be around the corner.

Although these memes address physical health and personal reflection, nothing is said about work, education, achievement, interpersonal relationships, or recreation. They illustrate how our experiences can cause us to focus on certain memes, pruning out what we think is irrelevant and honing in on one aspect of life. In this case, Student 2 has likely experienced or witnessed significant physical pain or illness, which narrowed her perspective. Consequently, the few rules that she chooses to live by are all within the context of physical pain and death. Such a narrow focus can be problematic; it is neither beneficial to approach every situation from this perspective nor wise to neglect other aspects of life.

If, when you do this exercise, you find yourself writing a similarly terse and limited set of memes, it may serve you to dig deeper. What experience caused you to view the world from this perspective? What memes are missing that might be beneficial to bring back into the mix? How do your rules and your fixation on the particular topic at hand affect your everyday behavior, thoughts, emotions, and reactions? Answering these questions will help you to rework your memes.

Student 3:

- Never stop believing in imaginary things
- You don't need a man to be happy
- True friends are always together in spirit
- Be a good camper (this means—be adventurous, try new things, and don't get grossed out easily)
- There is no such thing as normal—difference is the rule, not the exception.

As a whole, these memes are imaginative and idealistic. A significant value is placed on childlike wonder, particularly in the first meme, "Never stop believing in imaginary things," and the fourth, "Be a good camper." The last meme, "There is no such thing as normal—difference is the rule, not the exception," places an emphasis on the importance of acceptance and being nonjudgmental. Such open-mindedness about what is "normal" and the emphasis on not being constrained is echoed in the second meme, "You don't need a man to be happy," which states that the traditional path for a woman of finding a husband is not the only path to happiness. The third meme, "True friends are always together in spirit," places a large value on friendship, perhaps even more than on marriage when combined with the meme "You don't need a man to be happy." A countercultural, rebellious theme runs throughout these memes. They are also constructivist—they tell Student 3 that reality is based on her own perspective.

The memes, "You don't need a man to be happy," and "True friends are always together in spirit," provide guidelines about how to prioritize interpersonal relationships. While not intrinsically negative, if these memes were deeply internalized their devaluation of romantic relationships could result in difficulty maintaining this kind of relationship. This set has a heavy dose of reflective and psychological memes that provide an overarching life philosophy—"Never stop believing in imaginary things," "Be a good camper," and "There is no such thing as normal." "Be a good camper" could also be interpreted as a guideline for how to spend recreational time. However, it says nothing about fitness, health, achievement, work, or academics.

If Student 3 struggles to find direction in her academics or career, or if she has difficulty maintaining romantic relationships, understanding how her memes are affecting her choices in life could allow her to reevaluate the rules she lives by.

Student 4:

- Hard work is an absolute goodness
- Seeing perfection
- Attention to details
- Loyalty to hygiene and cleanness
- Taking a bath every night is a basic necessity for human sanitation
- Respect to seniors
- Punishments fall on you when you don't respect your ancestors
- A mega earthquake and tsunami will happen again soon.

The memes "Hard work is an absolute goodness," "Seeing perfection," and "Attention to details" are all related to the achievement domain of functioning and can be applied to academics or work. These statements teach the importance of a strong work ethic and of being detail-oriented. The next two memes, "Loyalty to hygiene and cleanness," and "Taking a bath every night is a basic necessity for human sanitation," are physical health guidelines that emphasize the importance of physical cleanliness. "Respect to seniors" and "Punishments fall on you when you don't respect your ancestors" both deal with interpersonal relationships. The message here is that respect within relationships is of the utmost importance, particularly respecting elders. "Punishments fall on you when you don't respect your ancestors" also has a psychological aspect to it—the statement has a "What goes around, comes around" philosophical tinge to it. Finally, "A mega earthquake and tsunami will happen again soon" also fits within the psychological domain of functioning. Here, the message is to expect disasters and negative events in life.

What is not mentioned in this set of memes is how to spend free time or how to attain personal happiness. Abiding by this set of rules could lead to an "All work and no play" lifestyle, and one that might not prioritize personal reflection. In contrast, the popular American meme, "Work hard, play harder," encourages a very different lifestyle. These memes also contain a pessimistic element that focuses on punishment and negative life events.

If Student 4 were to find herself generally unhappy, struggling to connect with her deeper emotions, or overwhelmed with work or academic commitments at the expense of time to relax, she may find it helpful to introduce new memes into her repertoire that give her some guidance for her free time and personal happiness.

Student 4's memes are another good example of memes heavily influenced by culture. The emphasis on hard work, perfection and details, hygiene, and respect is reminiscent of Japanese cultural values. Indeed, Student 4 is from Japan. The final meme, "A mega earthquake and tsunami will happen again soon," is another instance of a traumatic event that narrows focus and perspective. The 2011 earthquake in Japan likely brought the possibility of future disasters to the forefront of Student 4's mind, such that this is now one of the forces guiding how she lives her life. It is easy to imagine how such a mindset would affect Student 4's approach to life.

Student 5:

- Be polite, humble, respectful and smile at the world
- It's better to regret something you have done than something you haven't done
- Stay thin and always look your best—a good first impression is essential
- Hard work is the key to success.

The first meme, "Be polite, humble, respectful and smile at the world" is primarily an interpersonal meme; it prescribes how she should present herself to other people. The second, "It's better to regret something you have done than something you haven't done," is an achievement meme. It encourages seizing all opportunities, and it teaches that, in doing so, Student 5 will live a happier life than if she passes up experiences. "Stay thin and always look your best—a good first impression is essential" instructs her in both the interpersonal and health domains. What other people think is important, and the way to make a good impression is to stay slender and be physically attractive. Finally, "Hard work is the key to success" is an achievement-oriented statement that promotes a strong work ethic.

Compare Student 4's traditionally Japanese memes to Student 5's memes, which are much more in line with traditional Western values. The major emphasis within this set of rules is being polite, appearing friendly, seizing opportunities, working hard, and being thin. These values are often considered important for women in Western cultures, including America. The predominant message in these memes is that appearance is of utmost importance—be polite, smile, and look pretty. Looking good is emphasized more than being good.

These memes lack a rule about enjoying free time or achieving personal happiness and self-fulfillment. They give no spiritual guidance on making sense of life. Instead, the rules focus on relationships with others. There is also very little about how to achieve physical health other than staying thin, which may not actually promote healthy behaviors. The emphasis is more on looking good than on being healthy. While these values are not inherently negative, living strictly by these rules could produce maladaptive behaviors, such as a preoccupation with physical appearance, an over-commitment due to the need to seize all opportunities, and putting energy toward impressing others rather than personal happiness.

Student 6:

- Self pride stinks
- What happens in this house stays in this house
- It is what it is.

Student 6's memes are another good example of a terse, limited set of rules. "Self pride stinks" and "It is what it is" are primarily psychological memes about how the world works and how to behave in that world: Do not be narcissistic, and do not believe you can do much to change your circumstances. "What happens in this house stays in this house" is a rule for how to handle interpersonal relationships; the emphasis is on loyalty and secrecy. These memes lack anything about achievement, physical health, recreation, or achieving personal happiness.

This set of memes does not encourage deep exploration of situations, experiences, or conflict. Instead, these memes place emphasis on steadfast acceptance and loyalty. Imagine that these were the sayings that your parents repeated to you; what kind of message would they have been sending? One sentiment is clear—don't air our dirty laundry. When we read these, we get a feeling of a strict, authoritarian household where children are encouraged to obey and accept rather than explore and ask questions. The resulting limited, tough set of rules for Student 6 could significantly affect her self-confidence; her ability to express herself, explore, and ask questions; and her motivation to create change.

Student 7:

- Clean and mended
- Sit like a lady
- If you want something done right, do it yourself
- Who was your servant this time LAST year?
- Don't lie; someone will find you out
- Crying doesn't help
- No one has ever died of overwork
- Don't fight; don't argue.

The first and second memes, "Clean and mended" and "Sit like a lady," promote hygiene and a neat appearance, which can fit within both the physical and interpersonal domains of functioning. The message tells her to keep physically clean and to look nice for others. The memes "If you want something done right, do it yourself," "Who was your servant this time last year," and "No one has ever died of overwork" all refer to the achievement domain. Each of these rules promotes working hard, independence, and not relying on others to get things done. "Don't lie; someone will find you out" is interpersonal—the statement does not teach the moral lesson of being truthful, but rather the social embarrassment she risks if she should lie. The unspoken element is that others will think less of her if they catch her lying. "Don't fight; don't argue" is again interpersonal, as it teaches how to relate to and behave with other people. Finally, "Crying doesn't help" addresses the psychological domain of functioning by teaching her to keep a stiff upper lip and not to express her emotions. Recreational, personal happiness, spiritual, and physical health guidelines are all missing from this meme set.

In contrast to Student 6's concise list of memes, some of us will come up with numerous family rules to live by. For example, Student 7 was asked to submit three to five memes, and instead submitted eight. Although a lengthier list may seem more complete, it is not always the case.

Often, too, the memes in a single family are contradictory. While this can create some tension and confusion, it also allows family members to pick and choose the rules they adopt as their own. Student 7's list has some competing themes. On the one hand, the memes "Clean and mended," "Sit like a lady," and "Don't fight; don't argue" emphasize traditional female gender roles, appearance, and manners. However, some of the other memes contradict this, such as "Who was your servant this time last year?," "Crying doesn't help," "If you want something done right, do it yourself," and "No one has ever died of overwork." These emphasize self-sufficiency, keeping a stiff upper lip, and hard work, which are values encouraged in traditional male gender roles. Such conflicting messages are commonplace. We are constantly bombarded with a myriad of messages, values, and rules. It is up to us to select the memes that we live by.

Ultimately, it is up to each of us to determine what significance our memes hold. The important thing is to take an honest look at the rules that unconsciously influence our behavior, thoughts, and emotions, and to understand not only how they affect our present and future life, but also where they came from. In doing so, we gain the power to understand ourselves on an even deeper level and to change those unconscious processes that do not serve us well.

Slips

Have you ever said one thing, but meant another? These slips of the tongue, or "Freudian slips," are familiar to most of us and are the most commonly known form of parapraxes, or unintentional errors. A humorous illustration of a slip can be found on a popular coffee mug sold in the United States: "It's like when you say one thing but mean your mother."

Parapraxes are not limited to verbal speech; unintentional errors in memory or physical action also fall under this category. They include mishearing, misreading, mislaying and losing objects, and inadvertent physical gestures, among others. Although they are sometimes just an error, they may reflect a repressed motive, thereby revealing information about one's unconscious desires and thoughts.

In order for our slips to help us analyze our unconscious, we must notice and remember them, which is not easy. They occur within split seconds, and—by their very nature—are out of conscious control. Often we only notice that we have slipped when those around us look incredulous or start laughing at what we have said. Still, practice helps us recognize them. Try to keep track of your own slips. Pay attention to what you inadvertently say, write in emails, or do, and write these errors down so that you have them later for analysis. You can begin to look at patterns within your unconscious mistakes. Remember, too, that not all errors are slips—sometimes we genuinely just misspeak. You should examine the error within the context of your life in order to determine whether or not it is a true slip.

It is usual not to notice slips, because they are over so quickly. You may need those close to you on alert that you are collecting them, because as I said above, they may notice them long before you do. One of the key reactions in other people witnessing a slip is surprised laughter.

Once you have recorded your own slips, you can begin to analyze and interpret them. In order to demonstrate what this process looks like, let's look at a few famous and personal examples, as well as some from my students.

Having just stopped smoking a week prior, a man said "Pass the ashtray" at the dinner table, when he meant to ask for the beans. What do you think of the fact that he asked for an ashtray instead of the beans? Do you think this is a meaningful, significant error? What do you think it might indicate about his unconscious desires?

In the context of him recently quitting smoking, it was likely a true slip, rather than a meaningless error. He may have had every conscious intention of asking for the beans, but his unconscious desire and craving to smoke was so strong that it motivated him to say "ashtray," instead of "beans." Just before voicing this slip, he had declared with pride that he had not smoked in over two weeks and that he felt in control of his withdrawal. He did not want to "appear weak." This error in speech is a bridge between his conscious and his unconscious, providing a window of insight into what he may be repressing—his longing for a cigarette. He was trying to "be good" and conceal his desire for a cigarette, but it leaked out when he failed to monitor his stream of consciousness carefully.

There are generally two layers of content in slips: the manifest content, which is the straightforward subject matter (Pass the beans—I am over smoking), and the latent content (Not so fast; pass me the ashtray, the cigarettes, and the matches please), which is the underlying meaning. When analyzing slips, we look for both layers. We look for the double meaning. Usually one thing is said, and another is inferred.

Typically, both the manifest and latent content are true, though the manifest content tends to be more socially acceptable. In this case, the man probably did indeed want the beans and to quit smoking, which is the socially acceptable manifest content. However, another, deeper part of him also wanted the ashtray in order to smoke another cigarette, which is the less acceptable, unconscious latent content. Contradicting manifest and latent contents indicate that we have unresolved conflicting impulses. When we pay attention to our slips, we can bring these conflicts into our conscious work space and resolve them: Am I going to start smoking again, or be done with it?

These two layers are not always obvious. Sometimes, we defensively block the latent meaning, as did the writer of this newspaper headline: "Prostitutes Appeal to Pope." This story was about female sex workers having an audience with the pope, seeking some kind of forgiveness or betterment. That is the manifest content. The second, inferred meaning is that the pope is attracted to women who work in the sex trade. That is the latent content. Usually, when I discuss this headline in class, the students' reactions are mixed. Some read only the manifest content, and others immediately see the latent interpretation, which is usually given away by their giggling. However, not everyone who interprets the latent content finds it humorous. On one occasion, I had a nun in the class who did not find the headline funny at all. She immediately recognized the latent content and, due to her profession and firm beliefs, had a strong negative reaction to it. The headline also demonstrates how a slip can present in manners other than verbal speech: How we interpret other people's speech and actions, including what we hear or don't hear, can all fall under the category of slips and can tell us about our unconscious motives.

In 2007, the former president George W. Bush gave us another example of a verbal slip: "The best way to defeat the totalitarian of hate is with an ideology of hate—excuse me—with an ideology of hope." When we consider his history of aggressive reactions to Saddam Hussein, we can reasonably believe that this was not a meaningless error of speech, but rather a reflection of how he really felt. His stubborn insistence that there were weapons of mass destruction despite all evidence to the contrary demonstrates how powerful unacknowledged convictions can be—in this case, his belief in an ideology of hate.

Slips are not limited to words; they can be errors of behavior as well. One Sunday, a young, attractive woman came to church for the first time. Due to her somewhat inappropriate attire, she received many disapproving looks from members of the congregation. After the service, she approached an older woman, an established member of the church, presumably to introduce herself. As the young woman stretched her arm out to shake hands, the older woman—instead of greeting and welcoming the young woman—reached out and handed her a Bible. The young woman looked bewildered, and the older woman apologized, quickly put the Bible in her other hand, and then shook the newcomer's hand. We can infer that the act of giving her a Bible indicated how the older woman felt about her appearance and attire. Since it would have been socially inappropriate to openly acknowledge these feelings, she repressed them. Her true feelings then came to the surface in the form of a nonverbal slip.

Sometimes, behavioral slips occur in the form of what we forget and what we remember. One of my students recently started a new job in which she works at two different sites. She reported the atmosphere at one site to be very warm and welcoming, and the other more high-stress. Since starting the job, she had accidentally locked herself out of the stressful office three times, and zero times at the welcoming office. While this student admitted that the stressful office was not her favorite place to be, her professionalism required her to put these feeling aside. However, her negative feelings did not go away. Instead, they manifested as a behavioral slip—locking herself out of the stressful office. This student had no conscious intention of locking herself out, but her unconscious made clear that she did not want to be there.

While this student was aware of her true feelings about her work sites, this may not be the case for all of us. Sometimes we commit slips—be they verbal, written, or behavioral—and have no conscious awareness of why, or even that we have done so. If we pay attention to this kind of mistake, the small daily errors that we often write off as meaningless can actually lead us to our true unconscious desires, thoughts, and feelings.

In the end, we are each in charge of deciding what our own slips do and do not mean. In the case of the slip at church, only the older woman knew how she truly felt about the younger girl and why she handed her a Bible instead of shaking her hand, and only you will know if an error in an email is a typo or a meaningful slip with latent content. Only you can know what is personally meaningful, but in many cases, your slips are windows into your unconscious.

CHAPTER FIVE

Creativity and the unconscious: the objective correlative and the presence/hermeneutic dialectic

How art preferences can reflect your unconscious mind

"Art enables us to find ourselves and lose ourselves at the same time," stated Thomas Merton (1955). Or as Aristotle put it: "The aim of art is to represent not the outward appearance of things, but their inward significance." Most of us have experienced the feeling of losing ourselves in art. Some of us keep photographs of a beautiful sunset pinned up in our cubicles to calm ourselves amid a stressful workday; others listen to our favorite songs while driving home to buoy our mood after a rough day. Something about a piece, be it auditory or visual, resonates with us—we cannot use logic to explain why we are drawn to the piece, we just feel it. When it comes to art we are like sponges—we absorb a piece and transform its content into our own personal emotional experience.

Herein lies the power of art. When listening to a particularly gripping piece of music or contemplating a favorite painting, we stop thinking about what to make for dinner or about tomorrow's work presentation. Instead, these reality-oriented thoughts give way to an emotional experience that transports us. It is often this suspension of analytical cognitive activity and the wave of emotion that draw us to art.

Art encourages us to enter the default network state (discussed in Chapter Two), which acts as a bridge to our deeper emotions simmering below the surface. When contemplating a piece, our minds fall into this rest state and wander to past experiences or future constructions.

Successful art tends to be ambiguous, leaving a lot of room for personal interpretation. Depending on our own personal experiences and memories, each of us views a piece of art differently. An external stimulus or symbol can be transformed into a highly personal meaning by our own memories. When looking at Gustav Klimt's *A Field of Poppies* (1907), you may simply see a painting of flowers with no deeper meaning. However, when I look at this painting, I am immediately brought back to my childhood when I used to vacation with my family in a town with a similar field of flowers, very close to where Klimt actually spent his summers. The Attersee in the Austrian Salzkammergut, the Lake District, is where I had many coming of age experiences as an early teenager. And Klimt has always been an important artist to me because of his intense juxtaposition of the beauty and sensuality of women and their stylized robes full of enigmatic patterns, which are reminiscent of some genetic codes. When I see his painting, I am flooded with feelings of nostalgia, comfort, excitement, and peace.

This process is not limited to visual art, and can occur even more powerfully while listening to music. The connection between these musings and the art is emotional. While listening to Beethoven's famously melancholy piece, the first movement of the Moonlight Sonata, we may find our minds wandering to a sorrowful memory. Particular experiences in life are often tied to particular songs. Think back to your teen or young adult years when you shared a specific song, or a "love song," with someone. These songs become special markers for our amorous experiences and have highly personalized significance. They constitute yet another way to gain access to our unconscious emotions and mental processes that we may not be aware of. When we give in to the experience and allow ourselves to go wherever the art leads us, we suspend our thoughts of daily life and are able to access a deeper part of ourselves. In this way, we simultaneously both find ourselves and lose ourselves in art, as Thomas Merton so eloquently stated (1955).

Sometimes, we consciously select artwork or music that matches our mood. We are more apt to play Samuel Barber's *Adagio for Strings* when something reminds us of a missed loved one. Or we relish the mysterious power of the Sunrise movement in Richard Strauss' *Thus Spake Zarathustra* as we are getting ready to undertake a difficult task. The artwork we choose to engage in out of a myriad of possibilities can reflect our own state, both unconscious and conscious.

T. S. Eliot discussed the emotive quality of art in his essay "Hamlet and His Problems." According to his concept of the objective correlative, artists infuse their art with symbols of emotion that the viewer picks up on. The artist seeks to transmit to the viewer the type of state he or she is in at the time of the creation of the piece. What happens, Eliot theorizes, is a kind of emotional ping-pong between the artist and the viewer/listener, which uses the piece of art as a powerful vehicle. Remember how disquieting some of Magritte's paintings in Chapter One were?

Paying attention to how these pieces made us feel gave us insight into Magritte's internal landscape. Understanding these emotions and symbols within the context of his history allowed us to undertake a hermeneutic process of analysis and to interpret the specific personal meaning of these pieces.

Taking a deeper look at our own artistic creations can elucidate our own unconscious processes. Often when we create a piece, we do not consciously and deliberately choose each element of the image. Ideally, the process flows freely. When we enter this state of creation, we make unconscious connections between ourselves and what we put on the canvas. Analyzing our own creations for their emotional content within the context of our life is a powerful tool for shining light on our unconscious.

Sometimes, art is not personal and does not reveal anything about the artist. In the context of his childhood trauma, Magritte's early pieces, such as *Nude* (1919), are not particularly reflective of his unconscious; they are more like forced expected exercises for an aspiring painter. He paints and draws a classical theme, celebrating the beauty of the female body. There is not much hidden within these works, just a universal enjoyment of female nudity. It isn't until later in his career that he begins painting pieces under unconscious motives, filling his paintings with symbols, imagery, and emotions related to his mother's suicide. Gradually the unconscious theme seeps into his artwork and, as we saw from his statements later in life, makes him regret his preoccupation with violence and injury.

While an artist may not always intend to impart emotions through his work, he may still have unconscious motives that contribute to the piece and come through to the viewer. Consider how different the styles are between a typically complex and cognitive Salvador Dalí piece and a soft, gentle Monet painting. The artists may not have consciously planned the stylistic choices that appear on the canvas. Instead, the decisions about what to include in the painting, what to omit, and how to represent the images are often unconscious and reflective of the artist's internal structure.

Recognizing the psychological significance of our own artwork can be a tricky process. If we have difficulty seeing the emotional content of a piece that we have created, the piece may genuinely lack this layer of latent content, or our unconscious defenses may stop us from seeing the symbolic manifestations.

One of the most astounding examples of defenses distorting what an individual sees in a piece of art comes from one of my recent classes. When I asked a student to discuss the painting of Judith and Holofernes by Artemisia Gentileschi, she described how the two women in the picture were tending to the general's needs and soothing his pain. When directed to look at the dagger in Judith's hands, she described it as a cross, probably intended to help Holofernes heal. This is an excellent example of how our mind can play tricks on us and distort information about a beheading taking place when we have strong unconscious reasons to believe that women are not capable of performing such acts.

When interpreting a work of art, the first step is to sit with the piece and let it sink in, to see if any emotional leads emerge. Think about what is in front of you. Then follow your emotional reactions to the piece. Most of the time, you will find that you land somewhere—you will either like the piece or dislike it, it will comfort you or make you feel uncomfortable. You will have a sense of your overall impression. This emotional impression is what will tell you a lot about your unconscious mind. Sometimes, what we don't see in a work of art tells us more than what we do see, as in the case of my student above who did not see the dagger in Judith's hands. This hermeneutics process aims to bring rational thought and emotion together (see Burton, 2016).

Sitting with the piece lets in as much of the stimuli as possible. Then we can choose to follow the pathway of the emotional leads, or the pathway of rational thinking. A trained art historian would most likely choose the latter, describing the type of art, placing it into a temporal and historical context, and adding information about technique, the artist, and the public resonance with the piece. We encourage our students to follow the emotional route, letting the emotion evoked carry them to further detail and description and then trying to trim the entire package into a formulation, a narrative about what they see as important and touching in this art. Then we invite the class to add or subtract their thoughts and reactions. While there is much in common with what students report, there are also idiosyncratic elements in the responses, which most likely highlight some important fact about the person speaking.

The steps in the hermeneutic process while interpreting art (objective correlatives)

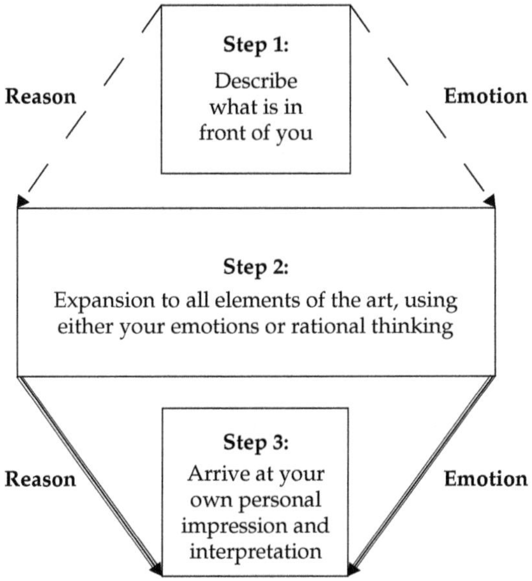

You can parallel this process by asking someone else what his emotional reaction is to the piece. If you are analyzing your own artwork, an unbiased viewer may pick up on symbolism and emotional depth that you, as the artist, missed. As in creative writing, metaphors usually add depth and texture to art that is not necessarily consciously controlled. Allowing ourselves to see these deep themes in art equally reveals unconscious processes, which can be uncomfortable or make us resistant.

Sometimes a lack of artistic proficiency is the primary obstacle to creating meaningful art. But we don't have to be artistically skilled or talented to use art to access our own unconscious mind. Instead, we can analyze the pieces of art that we are particularly drawn to. Often, when we enjoy a work of art, we resonate with the piece emotionally. Taking a deep look at the emotional content of a piece that we love can tell us about our own emotional state. When looking at a piece of art, each of us will unconsciously choose different aspects of it to focus on. Sometimes we don't even notice certain elements of a piece. Noting our own selections and omissions will provide valuable information about our unconscious mind.

This process is probabilistic rather than deterministic. When an artist paints a picture motivated by his unconscious emotions, we as viewers will not necessarily feel those exact same emotions. As Eric Kandel outlined in his excellent discussion of the neuroscientific underpinnings of art analysis, in the process of interpretation we access highly personalized information that is formed by our own experiences.

Likewise, relating to a painting does not mean that we have had the same experiences as those that motivated the creation of the painting. Just because we love Magritte's paintings does not mean that we must have had a traumatic childhood. Instead, the artwork leads us in a general emotional direction, and where exactly each of us ends up depends on our own past experiences and internal landscape. This is how the hermeneutic process works—we interpret a piece of art based on our own personally meaningful connections.

But the process is not completely idiosyncratic. More often than not, as I see in my class discussions, different people viewing a particular piece of art arrive at similar conclusions. The artwork leads most of us to a similar place, and it is in the final details that the discussion becomes highly personal and divergent. For many, the photograph on the next page would elicit feelings of calm and peace. Despite this common reaction, the specific memories and emotions each viewer has will differ. One person may fondly remember his recent vacation in Hawaii, while another may be brought back to a childhood trip to the beach with family.

Sometimes, this process will reveal previously unacknowledged feelings, which can be distressing and indicative of a past negative experience, as in Magritte's case. More often what it uncovers is much more benign, such as positive emotions, unconscious perspectives, or automatic behavioral patterns. We all have a repertoire of habits that we employ unconsciously and that affect our day-to-day experience. If we find ourselves stuck in a rut, repeating the same maladaptive behavioral pattern, we can gain some insight into the underlying motivations behind these behaviors by analyzing our art preferences or artistic creations. This gives us the power to make changes.

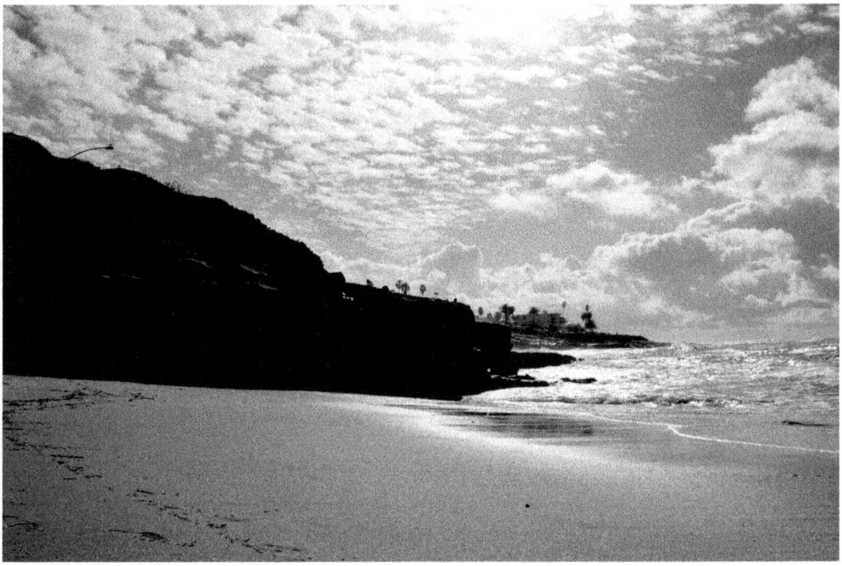

When analyzing our own artwork or art preferences, we may run into some obstacles. These techniques are often met with incredulity or defensiveness, particularly when they reveal unwelcome personal emotions or thoughts. Unless we have already undertaken some type of self-exploration and have developed a trust in following our emotional unconscious, these tasks may not flow easily at first.

We expect this resistance with each channel of access, but it may be particularly pronounced with art analysis. We are uniquely visual beings, and visual stimulation tends to be the most powerful for all of us. In order to overcome stumbling blocks, this technique requires our sustained interaction with the stimulus. We must sit with our emotions. When we do, this technique has the potential to reveal much more about us than memes or slips.

The measures of defensiveness that I discussed in Chapter Three can indicate how challenging interpreting a work of art will be for you. A high score on Repressive Defensiveness or Denial of Distress indicates greater resistance to unearthing one's deeper emotions. Because Denial of Distress allows for some conscious acknowledgment of negative emotions while Repressive Defensiveness pushes distress more into the unconscious, Repressive Defensiveness is typically the greater obstacle. Neither is insurmountable. Similarly, high scores on the REM-71 Factor 1 will often create difficulties.

Those who score below average in Restraint will encounter their own set of challenges with this task. Unearthing emotions that we prefer not to experience can be overwhelming and, without a certain amount of Restraint, can lead to behavioral outbursts. Working slowly and gently will help you approach this process.

To start this exercise, think about artwork you are particularly drawn to. Do you have a favorite painting, photograph, song, or dance? In the rest of the chapter I will focus on paintings and photographs. Have you created any pieces of art that really speak to you? Look for the ones that stir up your emotions. Look for pieces that you just love, even if you can't say why.

Once you have chosen a piece to work with, take a look at its manifest content, or subject matter. What is the painting of? What images does it depict? What colors are used? What is your first reaction to it? Is it uplifting or dark and dreary?

Moving into the latent content, or underlying meaning, of the artwork, you can begin to explore why you chose this piece. How does it make you feel? How does it affect you? What particular emotions or thoughts does the painting elicit in you? Do these emotions correlate with any specific aspect of your life? What aspects of the painting did you not notice or pay attention to on the first glance?

To pick up on this deeper meaning we must suspend rationality and follow our string of emotion, much like a patient in psychotherapy engaging in the process of free association. As Gordon Bower's experimental work (discussed in Chapter Two) has shown, strong connections are forged between seemingly disparate pieces of experience and memory, and these are tied together by their emotional feeling tone, not their logical progression.

When I look at the photograph on the next page of university students sitting on the grass in Vienna, Austria, for example, I feel a sense of sadness and nostalgia. The rationalist would say this does not make sense: the photograph is pleasant, not distressing or provocative. However, when put into the context of my own experience as a university student, my emotions make sense. I have fond memories of this time in life and have some sadness that I am no longer a carefree twenty-something sitting on the grass with my friends. This is the deeper latent content of the picture that we discover by following the emotional links.

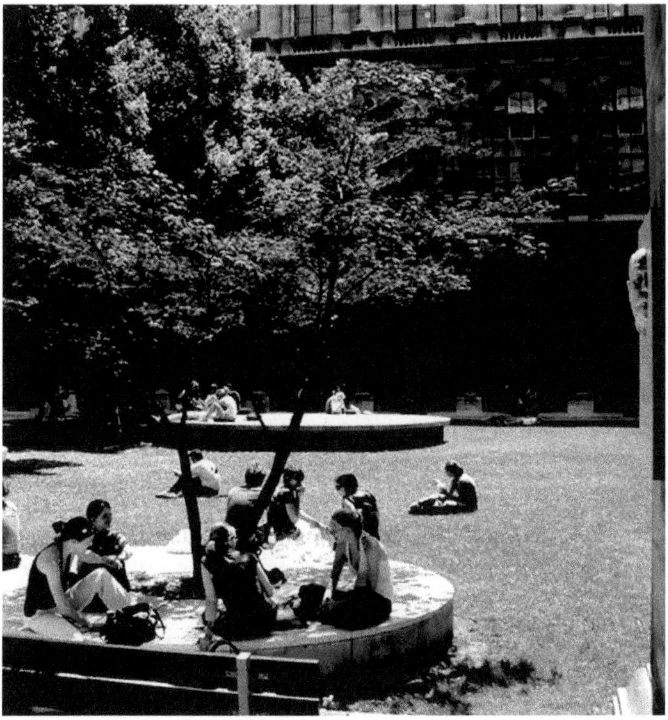

We can also access the latent content by guiding the search toward less obvious and more hidden aspects of the painting, uncovering contrasting or conflicting feelings and messages contained in the piece. Remember Magritte's *The Empire of Light* (1950) in Chapter One? At first glance, the scene is cozy and harmless. The blue sky, clouds, and the house look peaceful—the manifest content. But when we ponder the piece a bit, we notice some conflicting messages. Broadening the scope of inquiry, we notice elements of the picture that we may have missed at first, like the contrasting images of night and day. Most of us feel disquieted by this painting because the world depicted is not real. We do not live in a world where night and day coexist; this makes us uneasy. Again, we found the latent content by following our emotional reactions.

If this were your favorite painting, your interpretation of its meaning would depend on your personal experiences and psychology, and it would differ from that of someone else who likes the painting. One person may like it because he can relate to the feeling of uncertainty, confusion, and unease. Like the death of Magritte's mother, he may have experienced an event that made him question the dependability of his surroundings.

Another person may choose this as his favorite because he views life with a sense of wonderment and because he is drawn to surrealism. Rather than having a history of trauma, he may enjoy the infusion of mystery into everyday things; he enjoys contemplating the unknown.

Others might be drawn to the piece because they like the idea of changing their existing world into something very different; perhaps it speaks to their discontent with their current circumstances and reveals a longing for change.

Ultimately, a myriad of different interpretations could explain why we select this piece as our favorite, depending on our unique situation, experiences, and mental and emotional landscape. But usually there will be a common theme that emerges between different interpretations of a piece of art, and the details of those interpretations will differ according to personal memories. I encourage you to select the most salient explanation for why you relate to your chosen piece of art. With a certain amount of honest introspection, this selection will reflect your innermost, and likely unconscious, beliefs and emotions. In art, especially visual art, there are no norms. Our reactions are our own, once we let unconscious elements bubble up. While the art world may have standards that drive prices and subjects, you are your own standard.

As an example, here are two more of my favorite pictures. The first (on the next page) is a photograph that I took in Yosemite of a lake set against a granite rock formation in the background, which can also be seen as a reflection in the water. It is a serene, calm scene. Spending time in nature has always been important to me, and this manifest content very much resonates with me—remember my family meme of being a guest of nature?

However, the photo has a deeper layer of latent content as well. The crystal clear image of rock and trees in the water calls into question what is real and what is only a reflection. This concept is deeply ingrained in my life as a psychiatrist. When I work with a patient, my job is to decipher what is an account of his life that most people in his life would endorse and what is a reflection of his most idiosyncratic personal beliefs.

The scene takes place at sunset, which, while a beautiful time of day, also signifies that darkness is coming. The superficial emotional tone is one of calm and peace, but the impending night creates an undertone of threat. The absence of other humans and the potential for creatures such as bears, mountain lions, snakes, and coyotes add an additional element of threat. Having grown up in a family that survived post-World War II Austria, the perspective that dark times may always be on the horizon is one that has strongly influenced my life, as has the desire to overcome adversity and threat. Each of these ideas is also reflected in my memes, which we discussed in Chapter Four.

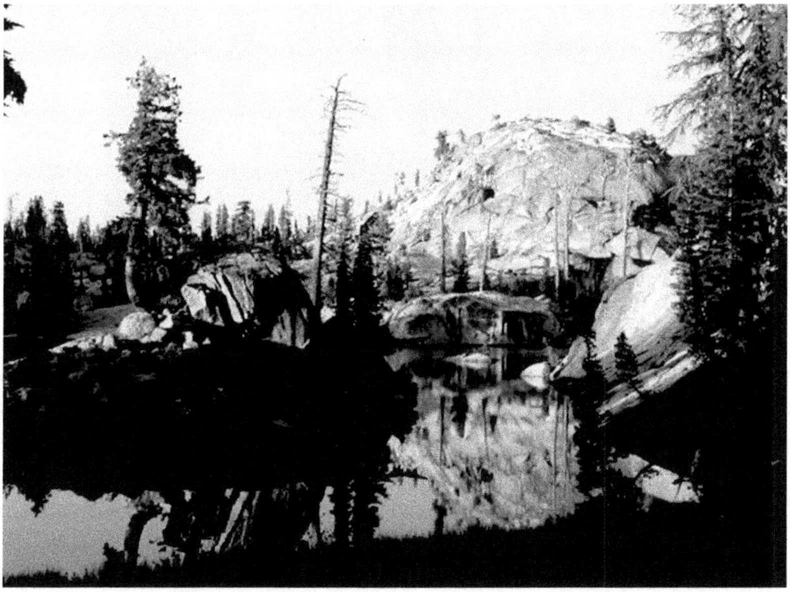

The second photograph (on the next page) was taken in Vienna, Austria and shows a traditional building reflected in the windows of a modern high rise. Again we see a reflected image, which highlights my interest in exploring the question of what is real versus our interpretation of reality. The collision of traditional and contemporary architecture is also a metaphor for emigration/immigration and brings up my experience moving from Austria to the United States. The latent content here is my desire to be in the U.S. and, at the same time, remain tied to my cultural roots.

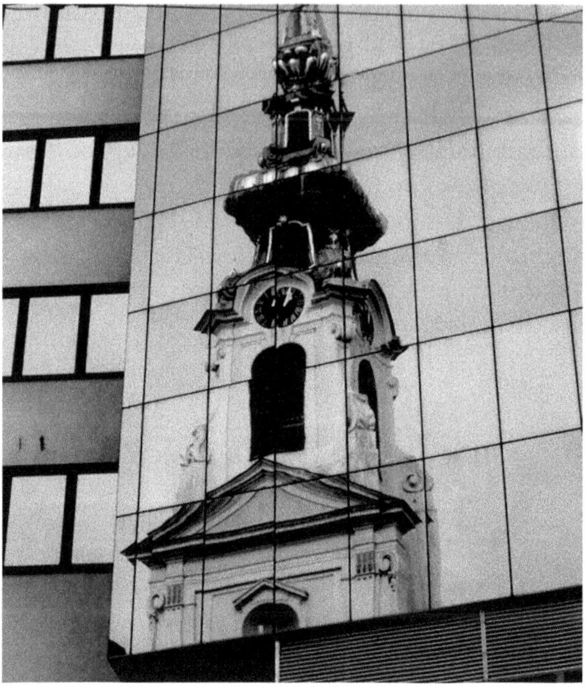

Sometimes the elements of a painting that we ignore or misinterpret tell us more about our unconscious than the elements we recognize. In one of my classes, Student 8 chose Arnold Boecklin's *Island of the Dead* (1880) as her favorite painting. It depicts a woman in a boat, floating toward a large island. In the boat is a coffin. This, in combination with the title *Island of the Dead*, leads us to conclude that she is going to the island to bury a loved one. The background sky is dark and ominous.

Student 8 explained that this was her favorite painting because it was such a pleasant Mediterranean scene. When prompted to further analyze the piece, she hypothesized that the woman in the boat was going to a picnic on the island. She had completely eliminated the coffin, and the meaning of the title, from her awareness.

Her omission of the central elements of the painting and misinterpretation of the image shed light on what she could have been repressing. I later found out that her husband had just been diagnosed with cancer, and his prognosis was unclear. So while her conscious, manifest mind wished for a picnic in a beautiful Mediterranean setting, her unconscious, latent mind simultaneously worried about her husband's future.

Now we will take a look at other examples from the class that are helpful illustrations of this process.

Student 9

Student 9 submitted NASA's photograph as her favorite piece of art. Taken with the Hubble Extreme Deep Field (2003/2004), it depicts galaxies billions of light years away from Earth, set against a dark, black sky.

The most striking thing about this photo is what is not there: no people, plants, or animals. In fact, there is no evidence of life at all, human or otherwise. What we see instead is an infinite mystery, an eternal unknown. This is a picture of a lonely, dark, cold place. There is no warmth of human contact here.

Student 9 is a scientist, so it comes as no surprise that she is attracted to a picture that highlights scientific discovery and exploration. This is the manifest content. There may also be an underlying layer of emotional latent content that draws her to this piece. Its interpretation will depend on her specific history, current circumstances, and personality.

If she finds herself feeling sad when contemplating the photo, her selection could reveal a feeling of loneliness or of being lost in some aspect of her life. Alternatively, if she feels calm and at peace, selecting this picture could be an indicator that she is more comfortable with space and science than with people and emotions. If she feels excited and energized, she may be attracted to mystery and intrigued by the thought of exploring the unknown—she could be someone who enjoys living on the extreme, challenging fears, and taking risks.

While I can demonstrate how to ask the guiding questions, it will be up to her to determine what the piece reveals about herself and how it is personally meaningful. The important point is to first ask the questions, what is and what is not in the photograph? Then follow the emotional links. Paying attention to how different pieces of the photograph make us feel will lead us in the right direction.

Student 9's psychometric scores (Chapter Three), were significantly greater than average for Distress, a measure of negative emotions (anxiety, anger, and depression), and significantly below the average for Positive Emotions (happiness and self-esteem). This suggests that she may have an underlying unhappiness with some aspect of her life.

At this point, she has a choice: Will she pay attention to her feelings and explore them, or will she try to let sleeping dogs lie? One way she can explore her feelings is to sit with her art selection and pay attention to what emotions come up and how they relate to her life circumstances.

Her psychometrics also provide information about how easy or difficult it may be for her to face these insights and emotions. Her Repressive Defensiveness score is significantly below average, and her Denial of Distress score is within the normal range. With lower than average defenses, she may already have some awareness of her negative emotions, and this process may come easily. Because she is not warding off uncomfortable and unfamiliar thoughts, she will likely be able to follow her own emotional trail to the deeper reason of why she selected this particular image as meaningful.

Because her Restraint score is significantly below average, this task may overwhelm her with a flood of emotion. Since this emotional activation can cause impulsive behavioral outbursts, she should approach the task slowly and with caution.

Student 10

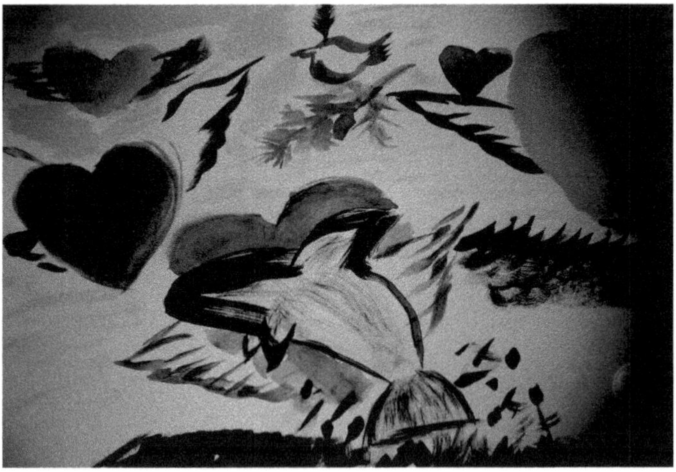

Occasionally I learn the motives behind a piece, allowing me to draw more specific conclusions about its meaning. The painting above, entitled *New Years*, is an original piece by Student 10, who submitted it as her favorite piece of art. It shows a black whale jumping out of blue water. Behind the whale is a pink heart with purple wings. To the left are two more hearts with wings, set against a bright yellow sky. To the right is what looks like a half yellow heart with one wing, and another pink heart. In the top center of the painting a bird sits atop a green branch.

The scene is not realistic; the different images in the picture are symbolic rather than accurate depictions. It is painted in a whimsical and simplistic style, yet contains complex themes and metaphors. It seems as if everything in the picture could fly away; everything is fleeting, especially love.

Student 10 explained that she painted this piece in response to a dream about a black whale that had beached itself because it knew it was dying. She felt unsettled by the dream and had a sense that she needed to help the whale.

At the time that she had this dream, her mother was going on a remote trip with little opportunities for contact, and Student 10 was feeling separation anxiety and insecurity over having to say goodbye to her. After the dream, she sat down to paint whatever came to mind in order to alleviate her anxieties, and she produced this piece. She recalled that she had tried to wrap the whale with love to heal it. However, the painting made her more anxious, because she interpreted the hearts with wings as floating to the heavens, which only heightened her fear of losing her mom. She now keeps the painting tucked away where she does not have to see it.

What is interesting here is that she chose a black, dying whale as the metaphor for her mother, both in the dream and in the painting. She did not choose a traditional symbol, such as a hen, or a cute fuzzy animal, like a rabbit. Instead, she chose a large, overpowering, black animal. She then painted hearts floating up to the heavens, an image that gave her anxiety to look at.

Student 10 could have some conflicting feelings about her mother that she does not like to consciously acknowledge but that bubbled up to the surface in this painting: On one level she loves her and does not want her to go, and on another, she sees her mother as a dark presence that she wishes would float away.

On the WAI scale, Student 10 scored highly in both Repressive Defensiveness and Denial of Distress compared to her age-matched norm. Her Distress and Restraint scores placed her in the Repressor category. Her high level of defensiveness means that she tends to avoid her feelings, particularly those that may cause distress. This fits with the interpretation that she may have some deeper, more negative feelings toward her mother that she does not wish to face. It is also not surprising that she put the picture away out of sight. Her Repressor nature wanted these feelings to be out of sight, out of mind.

Student 11

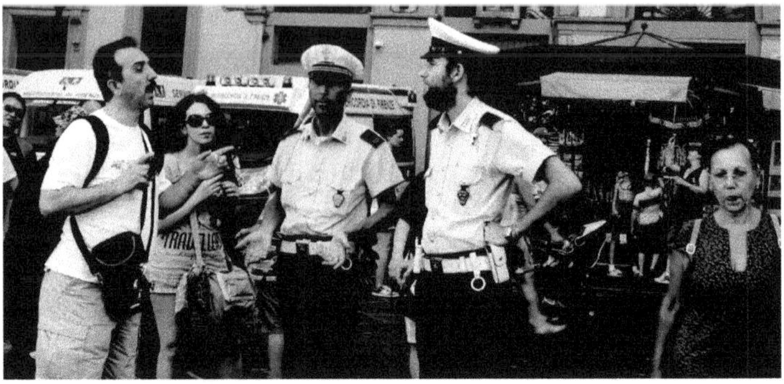

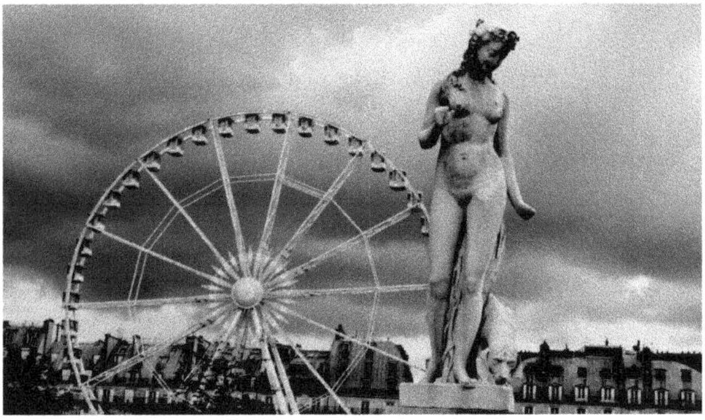

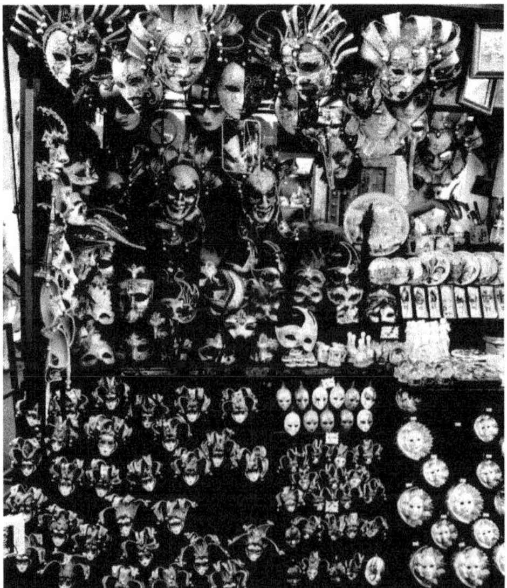

The three photographs on the previous page were taken by Student 11 and submitted as her favorite piece of art. In the first picture a man appears to be having a disagreement with two policemen. He is wearing a camera case and a backpack, and he is presumably a tourist. The two policemen look bored, uninterested, or fed up. The young woman with the tourist also looks irritated or bored. The second photo shows a female statue in the foreground with a threatening animal at her feet. In the background is a Ferris wheel, set against dark clouds. The third is a picture of a street vendor's stall filled with different masks.

These pictures are all photographs about traveling, being a tourist, exploring, and finding beauty in unexpected places. This is the manifest content. It is possible that Student 11 enjoys these pictures because she connects with these themes. Perhaps she enjoys discovering new places and has fond memories of trips abroad.

It is also possible that there is a deeper layer of meaning to these photographs—the latent content. When we look closely and sit with these pictures, we notice that each contains an element of threat. In the first, some kind of conflict takes place between the man and the policemen. It is easy to imagine that he is a tourist in a foreign land who got into some minor trouble. In the second, the clouds are ominous and the animal at the statue's feet is in a predatory pose. In the last photo, the masks do not look inviting. The emotional content of all three pictures is a feeling of unease and threat. If these photos reflect memories of some personal adversity, that could be the deeper element that Student 11 is attracted to.

Although Student 11 scored within the normal range on Distress, she scored significantly below average on Positive Emotions, a fact that could corroborate the hypothesis that these photos contain a layer of dark latent content. She also scored significantly below average on both Repressive Defensiveness and Denial of Distress. Her low level of defensiveness will likely allow her to explore the meaning of these photographs on a deeper level. Because she scored within normal range for Restraint, she should be able to do this exercise without being too overwhelmed by the emotions that arise.

Student 12

Student 12 chose *The Two Fridas* (1939), by Frida Kahlo de Rivera, a Mexican painter known for her self-portraits. In the picture, we see two depictions of Frida sitting and holding hands. On the right, she is dressed in traditional peasant clothing; on the left, she is wearing a white aristocratic dress. The hearts of both figures are exposed and connected by an artery that runs between them. The aristocratic figure is clamping the end of the artery with a surgical instrument. Blood drips onto her white dress, and black clouds lurk in the background. The peasant figure is holding a picture of Frida's ex-husband, Diego Rivera.

The lower class and upper class depictions of Frida in this painting are two sides of the same coin—two versions of one self, tied together not by the brain, but by the bleeding heart. No matter how much wealth or accolades she achieved, the painting shows us that she maintained an emotional connection to her past.

The emotional tone of this piece is heavy and serious. The stormy clouds in the background, the stoic expressions on Frida's faces, the exposed hearts, and the dripping blood all contribute to a feeling of quiet intensity, like something bad may be about to happen. There is an air of fierce loyalty during troubled times, and a feeling of determination to get through whatever is to come, together. However, we must not forget that the two figures are both Frida. The message is one of personal strength, determination, resilience, and maintaining a strong personal identity.

This message may be the latent content that attracts Student 12. We might expect her to place a high value on her strong sense of self, regardless of where she is, what circumstances she finds herself in, or what stormy clouds appear. We might also hypothesize that Student 12 feels a strong connection and sense of loyalty to her past.

Interestingly, at the time Student 12 submitted this piece as her favorite art, she had recently moved to America from Mexico and was adjusting to life in a foreign country, without friends or family. The painting could reflect her desire to maintain her Mexican cultural identity and connection to her homeland while living abroad. Moving to a new country alone can be emotionally tumultuous and taxing, which could be the underlying symbolism of the ominous clouds. Being here without any family or friends, it would make sense for her to feel determined to be strong and self-reliant, and to persevere through these challenges on her own.

When you approach this analysis for yourself with your own piece of favorite art, remember to ask yourself the three main questions that I have demonstrated here: What do you see, what do you not see, and how does the piece make you feel? Sit with the piece, let it take you down your emotional river, and then reflect on what circumstances within your own life may be associated with the feelings that come up. The emotional content will be the strongest clue as to what the piece reveals about your own unconscious processes. And as a final reminder: You are completely responsible for and in charge of your final formulations. Although I always have theories and thoughts about the latent content of what a student describes as a reaction to a piece of art, I in no way claim that I am always right in my assumptions. I do have a lot of experience in this process, but that does not make me always right. Only some of the time.

CHAPTER SIX

Expressive writing and the motivational unconscious: recreating and reconstructing the richness of your life

"Language ... is a means not only for representing experience ... but also for transforming experience," said Johann Gottfried Herder (1827). He is the originator of the thought that language is not only a way to communicate and describe, but a powerful tool to shape and transform. Telling stories is a way to bind together experiences, memories, and people. From nursery rhymes to literature, from movies to mythology, storytelling is everywhere; it is an almost universal property of languages across the globe and a skill that we develop as early as two to three years of age. One form of storytelling, expressive writing, does more than entertain the audience—it has been associated with a slew of positive effects for the writer, such as improved relationships, less negative affect and intrusive thoughts, more positive affect and working memory, and even an improvement in asthma symptoms. This has been shown largely through the extensive studies of James Pennebaker from the University of Texas at Austin.

In retelling our experiences and shaping them into stories, we don't just recite facts, we spin the events according to our personal views and infuse our memories with emotion. Consequently, what we remember about an event is not necessarily the same as what actually happened (see "The War of Ghosts" in Chapter Seven for a good example of this phenomenon). This is what Herder was referring to, as indicated by the quote at the beginning of this chapter.

Austrian philosopher Ludwig Wittgenstein attempted, and failed, to prove that language is a completely logical system that represents reality in his book, *Tractatus Logico-Philosophicus* (1922). Instead, as he came to realize later in life, we use language as a tool, organically grown out of our experience, to shape our experiences according to how we feel—and sometimes how we think—they should be. It is this emotional construct of reality that we want to access through expressive writing, because, as with the visual arts, a great deal can be learned about who and what we are when we systematically approach storytelling, writing, and journaling. As we have seen in Chapter Two, thinking about our autobiographical memories, telling them, and writing them down in more or less raw form is one of the access paths to the default network.

As discussed in Chapter Five, art speaks to us so powerfully because most humans are exquisitely visual beings. However, I hope to convince you that remembering our lives, describing events, and shaping them into narratives is as powerful, because it introduces a whole other dimension that art rarely exploits: time. By tying individual events into a string of events, we also make additional attributions: We assign causality. If A comes before B, then A most likely brings about B. This of course may be correct or incorrect, and this is what we exploit in psychotherapy.

In addition, as we create a memory and a story, we also do something else: We load the account with emotional charge—positive or negative. We link our senses and emotions with our expressive language system. We make sure that the listener/reader pays attention. We will discuss both these elements in greater detail in this chapter, and we will help you apply the insights of modern psycholinguistics to yourself (I am greatly indebted to one of my colleagues, Kristin Nelson, Ph.D., who helped me comprehend and apply much of what is to follow) (see Nelson, Bein, Ryst, Huemer, & Steiner, 2009; also see Nelson, Moskovitz, & Steiner, 2008).

The human tendency of modifying how we remember experiences most likely has a Darwinian adaptive value. It can be much easier to live in a happy, uncomplicated world than to be aware of all the dangers and discontent that surround us. (In Chapter Seven, when we discuss the retelling of dreams, we will include a very informative example of a girl telling and retelling a story, stripping it of all the frightening elements).

The price we pay by failing to face the dark side of life is that when things do not go well, we may not react appropriately. Changing one's lifestyle after a heart attack requires acknowledging the emotional trauma of the event. Cleaning up this memory may also cause us to ignore future warning signs of ill health. Sometimes, a traumatic event distorts memories in the opposite direction, leading to a continual negative perception of events. A heart attack victim with this tendency might subsequently interpret every physical symptom as a sign of a new major health crisis. Different people tell the story of having a heart attack very differently, and none would be exactly accurate. We discussed this in Chapter Three when we talked about the role of Repressive Defensiveness and Denial of Distress in our adjustment to stressful events.

Rather than consciously lying, we automatically and unconsciously distort the story, often in order to protect ourselves from difficult emotions, We skew reality according to our past experiences and, in doing so, deceive ourselves as well as others.

Before we continue to explore the world of expressive writing, let us spend a moment clarifying some of the terms, as they are not always applied in a uniform fashion. The table below summarizes the way these terms are applied in this chapter, based on the best consensus we can generate from the current literature.

Expressive writing, dictating, and speaking are different from other forms of creative writing. The goal is not to produce a well-crafted, polished story, it is to let our minds go and write down whatever comes up. The process is more like writing a stream of consciousness than writing a planned story. We follow emotional leads, not rational, logical ones. As I mentioned in Chapter Two, Gordon Bower proposed the idea that our brains file memories according to emotion. When accessing an emotion—feeling happy, for example—all our associations with being happy, including past experiences, are unlocked.

You want to get into the moment of whatever experience you write about and make it come alive, but be careful not to steer and plan. Let your emotional leads carry you where they may (Kris, 2011). This process is very similar to what Freud called free association—a definite misnomer. His thinking was more in line with Gordon Bower's research almost 100 years later that in fact writing or speaking like this is actually steered by unconscious forces. Free association is used in psychotherapy to help patients bypass unexpected roadblocks, recall events, and be creatively productive.

Terms and definitions.

Avoidance	A method of avoiding anxiety-inducing situations.
DAAP	The Discourse Attributes Analysis Program, a computer program used to measure referential activity.
Defensiveness	An automatic self-regulation process that we unconsciously employ when under stress. The process serves to keep us from conscious awareness of distress.
Event-specific knowledge	Vividly detailed information about individual events, often in the form of visual images and sensory-perceptual features.
Metaphor	A linguistic device that links two normally unrelated things in order to express an idea, usually phrased as "A is B."
Narrative	The linguistic representation of an event, experience, or story.
Narrative medicine	Medicine practiced with narrative competence and marked with an understanding of the highly complex narrative situations among doctors, patients, colleagues, and the public. Narrative medicine aims not only to validate the experience of the patient, but also to encourage creativity and self-reflection in the physician.
Narration	A recital of events, especially in chronological order.
Referential activity	Connecting nonverbal experience, including imagery and emotional experience, with words.
Simile	A linguistic device that explicitly compares two unlike things, often phrased as "A is like B."
Temporal junctures	The separation between two temporally ordered main clauses.

By following these emotional links during expressive writing, we gain access to the emotional construct of reality that we ourselves create. The process of storytelling allows us to begin to see how we might be distorting our memories and allows us access to emotions in our unconscious that we are not paying attention to. This process can help to digest, process, and put to rest even the most difficult of life events.

The part of the unconscious that we access with this exercise is known as event-specific knowledge—information about individual events from our past. This is a specific type of episodic memory, which is discussed in more detail in Chapter Two. These memories are uniquely time-stamped, vividly detailed, and can contain sensory, perceptual, emotional, and cognitive elements.

One uniquely beneficial aspect of expressive writing is that it is a permanent record. Once we have written it, we can continue to analyze its content without having to rely on our memory. Instructions for the exercise are straightforward. Sitting by yourself in a quiet, private room, safe from intrusions and distraction and with only your computer or paper and pen, write about a positive or negative event that has happened to you within the past three months. I encourage you to write continuously for the entire thirty minutes, without stopping or editing. Let the pen flow. You can start wherever you would like—at the beginning, midstream, or at the end of the event. The most important thing is to just keep writing.

If you cannot think of anything to write, continue to sit for the entire 30 minutes and write down whatever comes up. If English is your second language, I recommend writing first in your native language. Then translate your writing into English or have it translated, if need be. At the end of the thirty minutes, stop writing. Do not edit or correct your work. Try to write at least 300 words, but do not force yourself to do so. Three hundred words is roughly one to two double-spaced pages in most word processing programs. You may have to try several times to achieve this, but do not give up.

This will be a difficult task for some. The tendency to repress negative emotions may cause resistance and writer's block. A high level of Repressive Defensiveness, as measured by the WAI (Chapter Three), will make this task more challenging, as will a high Restraint score. A high score for Denial of Distress on the WAI could also cause the writer difficulty, but usually it facilitates writing. The process of minimizing the emotional importance of an event can, at the same time, decrease the resistance to writing about it.

Those trained in practices like mindfulness or yoga may also find this task difficult. These techniques teach us how to minimize the experience of negative emotions by taking our mind off the upsetting mental content. Expressive writing is different in that the goal is not to minimize immediate distress; the goal is to eventually feel better by allowing ourselves to first fully experience the emotions linked to a negative or positive event. It is almost a two-phase task: first we face what happened, then we work through it.

As I hinted in the initial paragraphs, in psycholinguistics, there are two writing qualities that are commonly used to assess a narrative—narration and vividness of speech. For the purposes of this discussion, I will define "narrative" as any account of an experience or event. A narrative is a story, however simple or complicated it may be. Stories are generally outlined with a beginning, which serves to orient the reader and set the scene; a middle, which presents a complicating action; and an end, which wraps up the story with a resolution.

Most people in my class can easily and intuitively determine whether or not a text reads as a story. Why should this be so? Given how early children's capacity to understand and then make up stories appears (usually happening between ages one and a half and five), we must surmise that this is due to some genetic programming which unfolds early in our growing up. Support for this idea also comes from linguistic research by Daniel Everett (2005) on the Pirahã tribe in the Amazon.

The Pirahã is a monolingual Amazonian tribe in northwestern Brazil that speaks a whistled, tonal, and sung language. The Pirahã language does not contain numbers or words for colors, and they do not have words that translate to "all," "each," "most," or "few." They do not linguistically combine thoughts into the same sentence (recursion). For example, they would not combine the two sentences "The man is running" and "The man is wearing a coat" into "The man who is wearing a coat is running." They also do not have a tradition of art, agriculture, myths, or religion. They do not speak or think abstractly. However, Everett showed that when shown the movie *King Kong*, the Pirahã understood the plot. Despite the extremely limited characteristics of their language, the Pirahã immediately, and without being led, understand the story—providing persuasive evidence that understanding storytelling is a universal human capability.

Without having tenses or a culture in which stories get told to children, without any sophisticated forms of sentence construction, when exposed to a Hollywood storyline, the Pirahã accurately summarized and followed the plot. Presumably, there is a native capacity in all of us that makes this possible. It is this native capacity which we want you to put to good use when analyzing your expressive writing exercises and, as we shall see in Chapter Seven, your dreams.

A note of caution: Daniel Everett's work has engendered a firestorm of criticism and counterarguments, mostly because his findings severely challenge the holy grail of language development (the language organ, as postulated by Noam Chomsky). Chomsky himself and many of his colleagues and understudies have attempted to discredit Everett's research for quite some time, and he has defended his findings quite effectively. If you are interested in learning more, there was an excellent summary in *Harper's Magazine* in August 2016 by Tom Wolfe. You can also refer to the 2007 article by John Colapinto in *The New Yorker*. The entire duel is actually another example of how in the scientific fields, especially those that are considered "soft," such as linguistics and psychology, there often exists a bias toward genetic explanations as a way to gain respect. Everett's work, though, which he has very effectively defended, is a great example of how culture and genes interact to produce complex phenomena. His work supports one of the major theses of this book, which I hope to have impressed upon you in Chapter Two: As we study increasingly complex phenomena, such as minds, motives, emotions, stories, and language, we are probably better served to explain them on the basis of a biopsychosocial model, where each level produces constraints and interactions, which then in the final analysis gets us closer to having a more realistic understanding of ourselves.

Now let us return to the task of analyzing your writing pieces. The first quality used to assess a narrative is "narration," which in linguistics refers to the temporal sequence, or the order and structure of a text. When we tell a story, we tend to order the events according to the time they occurred; first A happened, then B happened. This temporal flow also implies causality; if event A precedes event B, event B must have somehow resulted from event A. A text is considered to be a narration when it is temporally structured in this way.

The quantitative method of assessing the temporality of a narrative is complex, but one simplified version, created by Kristin Nelson, consists of counting temporal junctures. A temporal juncture is the separation between two temporally ordered main clauses. To find a temporal juncture, first parse out the main clauses. For example, "Humpty Dumpty sat on a wall, Humpty Dumpty had a great fall" would be separated into A) Humpty Dumpty sat on a wall, and B) Humpty Dumpty had a great fall. Next, reverse the order of the main clauses, and reread the text: "Humpty Dumpty had a great fall, Humpty Dumpty sat on a wall." Because this reversal changes the meaning of the story—in the first reading, Humpty Dumpty falls because he sat on a wall; in the second reading, he falls (presumably due to something other than the wall), and then sits on the wall—this is a temporal juncture. If the meaning remains the same when the clauses are reversed, it is not marked as a temporal juncture.

A piece with a high number of temporal junctures is likely to read like a story, with a sense of structure in the organization of events. A piece with a low number of temporal junctures is usually hard to follow, as it lacks a linear sequence of events. Later in the chapter, I will give examples of each of these types of texts.

An expressive writing piece that is structured and has a high number of temporal junctures indicates that the writer has somewhat processed the event. The author has thought about the event and digested it. He has packaged the experience into a cohesive story that makes sense and is easier to live with, particularly if it is a distressing, negative experience.

When the text must be written within a limited timeframe (e.g., when the instructions say, "Write for thirty minutes"), the number of temporal junctures must be corrected for word count. The formula is to divide 1,000 words by the word count of the text, which yields a correctional factor. That correctional factor is then multiplied by the number of temporal junctures found in the text. If the text length is limited by words, rather than by time—for example, if you select the first 300 words of a book—it is not necessary to correct for word count.

The mean number of temporal junctures for ages 12–75 is 11.1 per 1,000 words (+/– 12.2; scores outside the range of 5.0–17.2 are considered significantly different from the mean) for a free association text, and 16.0 per 1,000 words (+/– 12.8; scores outside the range of 9.6–22.4 are considered significantly different from the mean) for a text about a stressful event. We tend to structure negative experiences into more of a story than neutral ones.

The temporal juncture method is time consuming; one expressive writing text can take one to two hours to analyze. A quick and dirty method of assessing temporal sequences involves counting the words in a text. In general, the number of temporal junctures correlates positively with the number of words produced in a given time period: The more verbose the text, the more likely it is to contain a high number of temporal junctures. When using this method, adhering to a strict time limit is important in order to eliminate time as a confounding factor.

Increased time allows one to write more. In the examples throughout this chapter, I will use word count as a proxy for temporal junctures.

Using data from previous classes, I have found the average number of words written in thirty minutes to be 508.0, with a standard deviation of 406.5. Word counts that differ more than 0.5 of a standard deviation from the norm (i.e., outside of the range 304.7–711.2) are considered significantly different from the average.

Because the odds of producing temporal junctures increase with the number of words written, writing more will often produce more temporal junctures. Clearly, counting words is too simple a method to reflect the true complexities of narration. Even so, I have found word count to correlate about +0.6 with the count of temporal junctures: generally, when one goes up, the other goes up. Word count therefore does give some hint at this crucial construct.

Word count would produce a lot of error if used to analyze a text from someone who "blows hot air," or someone who fills the allotted thirty minutes writing meaningless or vapid words. While these texts seemingly fulfill the demands of the task by producing writing, in reality they evade the task by avoiding writing about the issues at hand. The second psycholinguistic measure, vividness of speech, addresses the content of the writing.

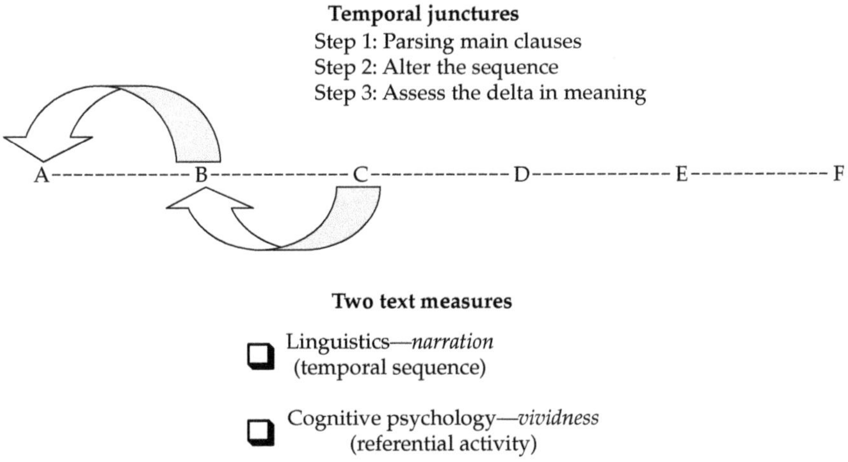

Vividness is a concept that comes from cognitive psychology. In a vivid text, the author accesses sensory and emotional experiences and, in turn, translates these experiences into words. In a highly vivid text, many, or even all, sensory input channels are linked with expressive language.

The writer paints a picture of an experience using descriptions of sound, sight, smell, touch, etc. Readers rate this writing as clear, detailed, concrete, and imagistic, as opposed to vague, abstract, or general.

The net effect is that the text takes us into the author's world. The language transports us—it evokes a corresponding imagistic experience in us as readers, and we feel like we are right there with the author. T. S. Eliot called this experience the objective correlative: by writing expressively and vividly, the chances are great that the author will make us feel the emotions that she intended to impart. This skill can be groomed and greatly improved with practice, and as we will see below, creative writers are in full command of this way of writing—when they want to be.

Psycholinguists developed referential activity in order to actually measure vividness. Referential activity refers to both the emotionality of a text and linking all our senses with expressive language, which can include detailed imagery (Mergenthaler & Bucci, 1999). This type of writing tends to feel emotional, with an experiential immediacy. It often suggests that there is an emotionally significant connection between the author and the text. When writing a vivid piece, the author must bring herself back to the experience or place that she writes about, and that typically involves reexperiencing the emotions of the event. Very often, the writer or speaker also shifts into the present tense. I have found that this occurs especially in patients recounting outright traumatic events. In recreating the scene, she lets the reader in, and we readers can pick up on that emotion and join right into the story.

Writing vividly, particularly about personal events, makes us vulnerable. Letting a reader into our private, internal world requires trust and confidence that we will not be judged. Extending that trust is unnerving for most of us, but it is likely to be an especially difficult task for those with high levels of Repressive Defensiveness and/or Restraint (Chapter Three).

One way to quantitatively measure the vividness of a text is with a program called the Discourse Attributes Analysis Program (DAAP), developed by Wilma Bucci and Bernard Maskit. It assesses the vocabulary of a text and produces an index called referential activity, which is a measure of vividness. Using transcripts of high and low emotionally charged texts, Bucci and Maskit (2006) created a dictionary of words that were assigned specific referential activity scores. The DAAP program compares the words within a text to this referential activity dictionary and gives each word a relative numerical weight. These values are then averaged to produce a mean referential activity score for the text.

Possible mean referential activity scores range from a minimum of 0 to a maximum of 1, with a neutral value of 0.5.

When I ask students to write a text for DAAP analysis, I suggest that they sit for thirty minutes and write on the given topic. With these instructions, I limit the time, but not the number of words. I tell them to aim for about one or two double-spaced pages, which is usually around 300 words. Texts that are much shorter than this are vulnerable to random error.

I then run about the first 300 words (ending on a whole sentence) of each text through the DAAP for analysis. This controls for the fact that a longer text will provide greater opportunity to be expressive than a shorter one. (Note: In psycholinguistics, referential activity scores are often corrected for word count in the same way as temporal junctures: 1,000 words are divided by the word count of the text to obtain a correctional factor. The correctional factor is multiplied by the raw referential activity, producing a corrected referential activity score. By selecting the first 300 words of each text, I do not need to use this technique. I have learned with experience that the first 300 words are usually an accurate representation of the text.)

The data produced by the DAAP program can also be used to generate a graph, like the one below. The horizontal X-axis represents the ordinal number of words in the text, while the vertical Y-axis represents the referential activity of those words. For example, at the X-axis point "100," the Y-axis value of the line gives us the referential activity of the 100th word in the text.

The graph is a visual representation of when the text becomes vivid. In the graph below, the text is most expressive in the middle (around word 145), when the line graph peaks. In these graphs, the neutral line is set at 0.5. So, if the referential activity line is above 0.5, the text is considered vivid; if the referential activity is below 0.5, the text lacks expressivity.

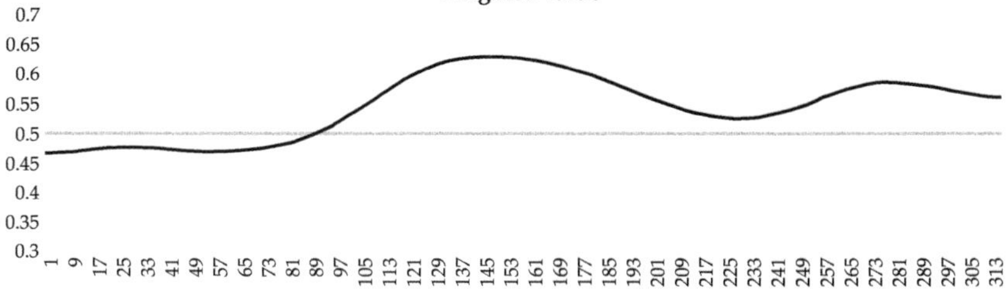

To get the most accurate results using the DAAP program, it is best to use texts that are around 300 words in length. Those shorter than 250 words create error and do not produce accurate referential activity scores. Because expressivity is difficult to sustain over a long stretch of writing, texts longer than 500 words usually produce a flattened graph. If some sections of a long text are referential and others are non-referential, the values will even each other out and produce a mean referential activity score that is in the average range, masking the expressivity of the referential sections. For example, the graph below corresponds to a 978-word story in which short sections are highly referential. The mean referential activity for the entire story is 0.52, a value within the average range. However, if I run the first 300 words through the DAAP, the mean referential activity shoots up to 0.58. The text contains sections that are highly referential, but the peaks and valleys over 978 words cause the overall mean referential activity to average out.

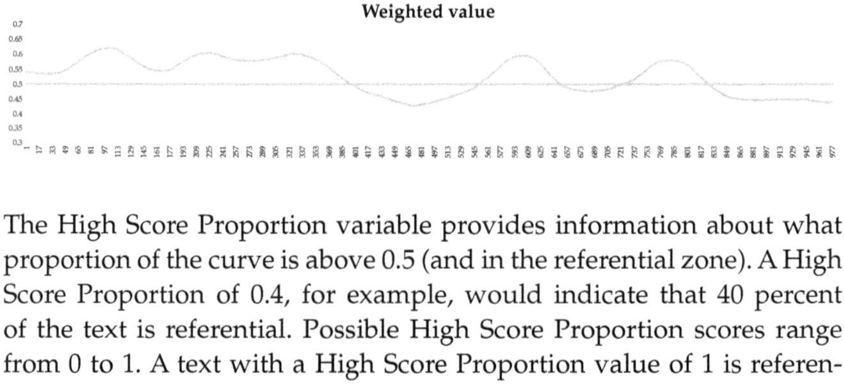

The High Score Proportion variable provides information about what proportion of the curve is above 0.5 (and in the referential zone). A High Score Proportion of 0.4, for example, would indicate that 40 percent of the text is referential. Possible High Score Proportion scores range from 0 to 1. A text with a High Score Proportion value of 1 is referentially active from beginning to end, and its line graph never dips below 0.5. A text with a High Score Proportion score of 0 does not contain any referential sections, and its line graph never goes above 0.5.

A High Score Proportion of 1 indicates that the text is referentially active, but it does not tell us *how* referentially active. The Mean High Score variable provides this information. The Mean High Score is calculated by taking all the points in the curve that are above 0.5, finding the difference between those points and 0.5, and then averaging those differences. In other words, this score indicates by how much the graph is above 0.5, on average. So, a text that produces a low Mean High Score means that even though the text may be referentially active, it is only slightly so. The corresponding line graph would only be slightly above the neutral 0.5 line. Conversely, a text that produced a high Mean High

Score is highly referential. The maximum possible Mean High Score is 0.5, which would require that every single word in the text scores the maximum referential activity value of 1. The minimum possible Mean High Score is 0. By definition, if a text has a High Score Proportion of 0, its Mean High Score will also be 0, because the line graph never goes above 0.5.

Referential activity, High Score Proportion, and Mean High Score norms for adults are listed in the table below. The last column of the table indicates the 0.5 standard deviation range above and below the mean; scores outside this range are significantly different from the average. In the sample used to calculate these norms, subjects were asked to write about a negative or a positive event. The two conditions were then combined to calculate these norms.

Adult norms across all conditions.

	Mean	*Standard deviation*	*½ standard deviation range*
Referential activity	0.53	0.04	0.51–0.55
High Score Proportion	0.61	0.37	0.43–0.80
Mean High Score	0.05	0.04	0.03–0.07

The same bell curve normal distribution that was discussed in Chapter Three applies here. Most people score within one standard deviation of the average. A smaller proportion of people score outside of one standard deviation.

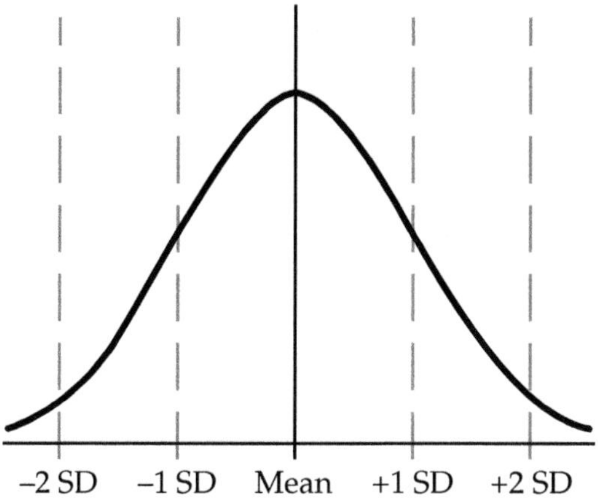

When a text produces a line that is sustained above 0.5 (with a High Score Proportion of 1), rather than one with peaks and valleys, its author has maintained a state of emotional connection with the writing. When the line fluctuates, the author is emotionally approaching and avoiding something within the text, either consciously or unconsciously.

Generally, mean referential activity scores above 0.5 indicate that the author is writing about something close to the heart, as opposed to close to the brain. She is allowing herself to experience and express a full range of emotions. The manifest content (discussed in Chapter Five) is referentially active. When the mean referential activity score decreases and the graph flattens out or dips below 0.5, the author is backing away from emotional content. At face value the manifest content may not seem particularly significant. However, the writing probably contains something of importance that the author does not want to get into. Her defenses kick in and prevent her from elaborating too vividly on this underlying latent content.

This latent content is what hangs around the unconscious and, unbeknown to the author, influences her thoughts, behavior, and emotions—the sleeping dogs that may be beneficial to explore more deeply. Where the referential activity increases and decreases throughout a text is an important clue about what may be hiding in the unconscious—thoughts and feelings that can then be teased out and addressed through further expressive writing exercises.

You may find more information about the DAAP and download the program at: http://www.thereferentialprocess.org/the-discourse-attributes-analysis-program-daap. It is a bit complicated to run, but it does provide extremely useful information. Over the years different versions of the DAAP have been released; we have worked with the first and current versions (DAAP09). If you are interested in downloading a copy, we recommend downloading the current version and staying up to date with program developments.

We have tested the old and the new versions, and we have been satisfied with very similar performance by both. In discussing these results with a mathematician and psychiatrist from the University of Vienna, Dr. Lukas Pezawas, he agreed with our current decisions on how to proceed. We are satisfied that there are no methodological impediments to working with the current version of the DAAP only.

For those interested in delving deeper into these comparisons, we are willing to work out arrangements where we can share data and discuss joint publications.

The unconscious data contained within expressive writing is sometimes wrapped up in metaphors, much as dreams are. Rather than universal, these metaphors and symbols are highly individualized: The same metaphor can have very different meanings for each of us, depending on our culture and personal experiences. To someone in the United States, a cross is a symbol of religion and salvation; to someone who has never had any contact with the Western world, a cross would be just two pieces of wood. To a Muslim, a cross may represent challenge or even threat. Metaphors and symbols take on an even more individualized meaning based on personal experience. Writing and telling stories utilizes metaphors and similes, but usually elaborates them—unpacking them, as it were. Poetry, by contrast, keeps everything tightly compressed at this very high level of communication.

The metaphor and its meaning provide valuable information about the latent content of a piece, but because the meaning of metaphors is so individual, a human brain is required for this step in the analysis. The DAAP does not typically detect the vividness of metaphoric language. Even though metaphors can be highly emotional, they are compacted, compressed emotion that the DAAP has difficulty recognizing. Poetry, for example, is highly condensed language rife with metaphors and hidden emotions, and it does not produce accurate DAAP results.

When a text meets the requirement to be a story (it has a beginning, middle, and end), a narration (it is structured in temporal sequences), and the language is vivid (there is a high level of referential activity), it is considered a balanced narrative. Not only are these texts generally the most captivating for the reader, but they are beneficial for the author. Packaging an experience into a structured, vivid story helps the author to reshape emotionally important experiences, process them, and move past them.

That is ultimately the goal of expressive writing. We may not instinctively write this way right off the bat, but with practice and time, the odds are that our expressive writing pieces will naturally become more structured and expressive. It is in this process that we find the psychological benefits. One of the functions narration serves in our lives is to stabilize disconcerting events and to help us understand what caused particular predicaments.

Mean referential activity and temporal junctures correlate positively with each other. When we vividly express our personally significant experiences, we tend to order them in a way that makes temporal sense.

This is usually easier to accomplish when writing about positive events than negative events, since our defenses can prevent us from delving too deeply into negative experiences.

Both mean referential activity and temporal junctures correlate negatively with high levels of defensiveness, meaning that defensiveness generally makes it more difficult to produce a high level of referential activity, temporal junctures, and word volume. In other words, a high level of Repressive Defensiveness creates more difficulty in accessing the emotions necessary to express an experience as a balanced narrative. When we are reluctant to access our emotions, we are less likely to bring the reader into our emotional world. This phenomenon is often experienced as writer's block. Those who classify as Repressors on the WAI (discussed in Chapter Three) will typically have the most difficulty producing a balanced narrative due to their high level of defensiveness.

Narratives, referential activity and repression

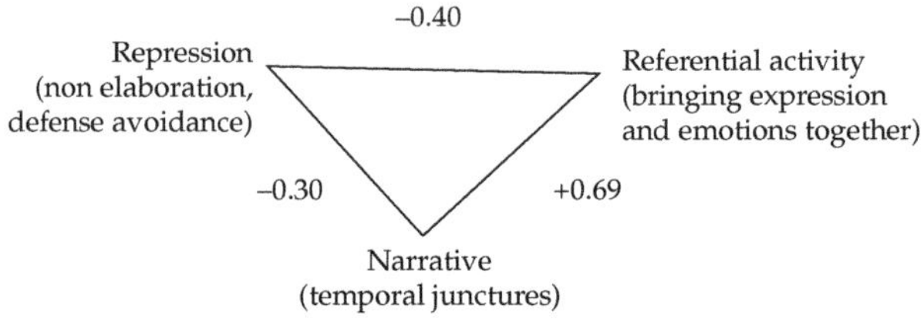

While mean referential activity and temporal junctures do tend to overlap, this is not always the case. We must think of the relationship between the two as more of a quadratic model, as depicted in the graph on the next page. This model recognizes four types of texts—Vividness, Synthesis, Movement, and Constriction. These labels, derived from clinical psychology and psycholinguistics, are by no means final at this time.

When a text scores high in referential activity but low in the number of temporal junctures, it falls into the quadrant I label Vividness. These texts contain a significant amount of emotional content, but they lack structure and order. Rather than telling a story, these pieces can be emotional overflow. While this type of expressive writing can provide a sense of relief, it lacks any sense of causality between events. Often in my class, I hear people say, "If I let it all out and just get my emotions out, is that what you want me to do?" While doing that does have some value and will unburden some emotion, writing that way doesn't necessarily lead to an understanding of why we feel the way we do.

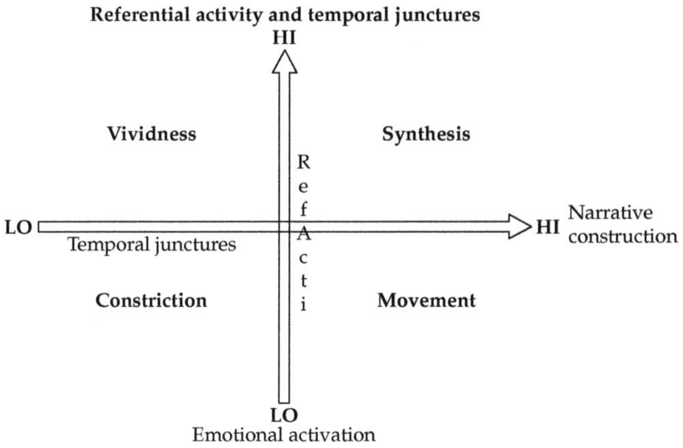

Texts that fall in the next quadrant, Synthesis, are high in both referential activity and temporal junctures. These pieces are both colored with emotion and temporally structured. They feel vivid and concrete, and they draw the reader in. By both expressing emotion and assigning some causality to the events, writing the story helps the author to process the experience and understand her emotions.

Alternatively, a text can be low in both referential activity and temporal junctures. I will label writings in this quadrant, Constriction. They have very little emotional content and they lack a clear structure. These texts can be vague, abstract, or outright minimalist. There is no story, no temporality, no description of events, and no expression of emotion. The author does not let you into her world. She probably feels some resistance, consciously or unconsciously, to expressing these experiences.

Finally, texts that are high in temporal junctures, but low in referential activity fall into the quadrant labeled Movement. In these pieces, the author clearly delineates the sequence of events, but provides very little emotional context. The text tells the reader what happened but says nothing about the driving emotions. This author does not get the full benefit of the exercise without getting into the nitty gritty of the emotions surrounding the experience, and likely has some psychological resistance to these emotions.

These classifications can also be applied to creative writing pieces. A story will fall into one of the four categories depending on the goal and strategy of the author. Some authors usually write with a particular, single style, while others switch quadrants depending on the goal of each story. In some of the excerpts below, for example, different stories from the same author fall into different categories. Each type of writing can be effective in eliciting a distinct experience for the reader; each type provides a very different objective correlative.

Similar to analyzing art preferences, what literature we are attracted to can give us information about our emotional landscape and unconscious. We select a piece of writing that we like because we resonate with the author's point of view. On some emotional and personal level, we agree with his perspective. That selection, in turn, tells us something about ourselves.

Let's look at a few excerpts from writers. I have selected the first 300 words (ending on a whole sentence) from a variety of different authors and run these passages through the DAAP program. Each of these passages has a very different strategy for pulling the reader into the story.

The word counts reported below are the number of words within each passage that contributed to calculating the mean referential activity score in the DAAP program. Because the DAAP referential activity dictionary does not contain all English language words, and because the program breaks up contractions into two separate words, this "DAAP Word Count" is often different than would be found by simply counting the words in the passage as they are written below (i.e., Microsoft Word's "Word Count").

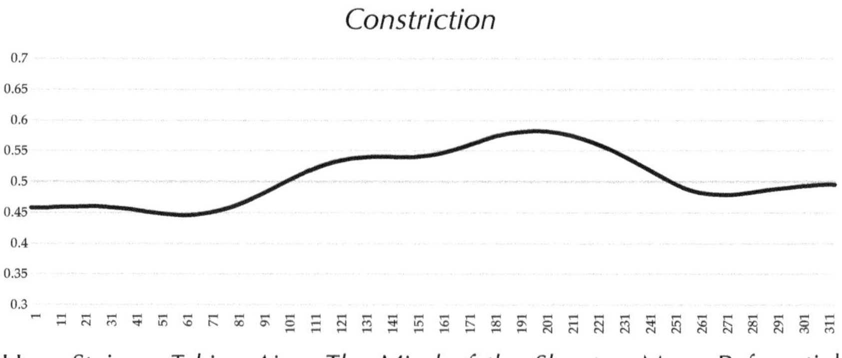

Hans Steiner: *Taking Aim—The Mind of the Shooter*. Mean Referential Activity = 0.51, DAAP Word Count = 319. High Score Proportion = 0.47, Mean High Score = 0.05

> Pretty cool title for a website, huh. You think I am joking. BUT I AM THE GREAT TIDE THAT WILL WASH ALL YOU TRASH INTO THE SEA! By the time I am done you will be dead or wish you were, because so much of you is hurting and missing and bleeding and screaming and shitting your pants. I will be in that next dimension waiting for you, and if you scum should make it to that your miserable little lives your pathetic being will not even be visible then. You will be blown away while I enter the greatest secret covenant with the Prince of Light who rules the universe and disrobes god the impostor. In this covenant I am cloaked in darkness and I can claim all the lives of those that have tortured me needlessly and cruelly. All I wanted was to give all of you of my greatness, bestow upon you the secrets of the universe, because I am the flame that ignites Armageddon, the final battle for supremacy where the Prince of Light, yes he will sweep away the weepy whiney masses, you fake Christians with all your love for your fellow man. Really, because all I wanted was to sit at your table in the breaks, all I wanted was to sit and be part. But you turned away and behind my back mocked me. I saw it, how you pulled your nose down to your lips, how you used a dust mop to mock my hair, how you hunched to show me sitting. If you are still alive then, I will enter your brains like a purple poison and make you yearn for the covenant, but you will be denied because you are the ones that truly are not worthy. You will be frozen in the vast pool of light swimming on top of an eternal cauldron of darkness and icy stillness.

When reading this piece, we have no idea where the story is taking place or who the speaker is. We can gather that the speaker is angry, but we have no idea why or at whom. Despite its obvious wrath, the writing does not elicit a strong emotional reaction from us as readers. We can recognize that the writing is about anger, but the stream of consciousness style does not make us actually feel the rage. This is reflected in a low referential activity score of 0.51. Even though 47 percent of the text is referential, that 47 percent is on average only 0.05 above the neutral line. The remaining 53 percent of the text is unreferential. The piece also lacks a logical, temporal progression of events. There is a palpable distance between the story and us as readers. I classify this writing as Constriction.

This story describes a school shooting that I did some research on. Whenever I get feedback about this story, people report an extreme reaction of alienation and a feeling of distancing from this character. They find him very hard to empathize with, do not understand him, and often dismiss him as "just crazy." This is indeed the impression I wanted to give of this shooter, who after shooting others killed himself.

Another even more extreme example of Constriction is the opening of Samuel Beckett's novel, *Molloy*:

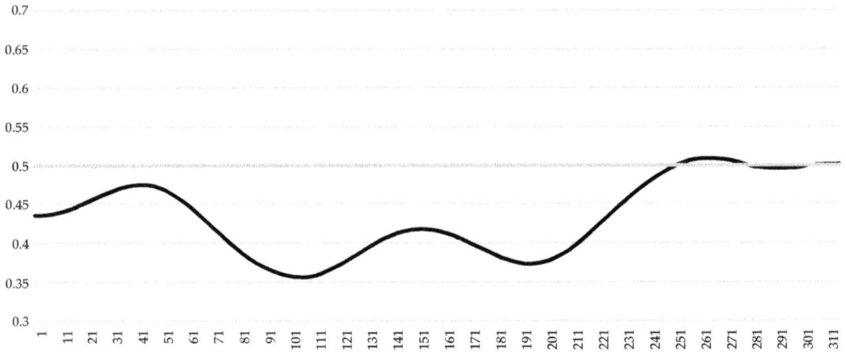

Samuel Beckett: *Molloy*. Mean Referential Activity = 0.43, DAAP Word Count = 318. High Score Proportion = 0.10, Mean High Score = 0.00

> I am in mother's room. It's I who live here now. I don't know how I got there. Perhaps in an ambulance, certainly a vehicle of some kind. I was helped. I'd never have got there alone. There is this man who comes every week. Perhaps I got here thanks to him. He says not. He gives me money and takes away the pages. So many pages, so much money. Yes, I work now, a little like I used to, except that I don't know how to work any more. That does not matter apparently. What I'd like now is to speak of the things that are left, say my goodbyes, finish dying. They don't want that. Yes, there is more than one, apparently. But it's always the same one that comes. You'll do that later, he says. Good. The truth is I haven't much will left. When he comes for the fresh pages he brings back the previous week's. They are all marked with signs I don't understand. Anyway, I don't read them. When I've done nothing, he gives me nothing, he scolds me. Yet I don't work for money. For what then? I don't

> know. The truth is I don't know much. For example my mother's death. Perhaps they have not buried her yet. In any case I have her room. I sleep in her bed. I piss and shit in her pot. I have taken her place. I must resemble her more and more. All I need now is a son. Perhaps I have one somewhere. But I think not. He would be old now, nearly as old as myself. It was a little chambermaid. It wasn't true love. The true love was another. We'll come to that. Her name? I've forgotten it again.

This piece is presumably about someone who is aging and dying—the manifest content. When reading the piece, does it bring up any emotions in you? Do you connect with the speaker? Do you have a clear idea of where the story takes place or what is happening? The net effect for the reader is a powerful feeling of alienation—even more so than with my Constriction piece above.

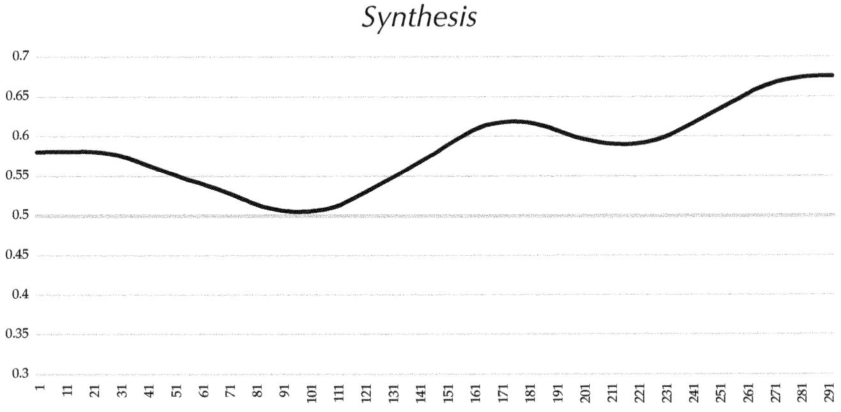

Hans Steiner: *Peripeteia*. Mean Referential Activity = 0.58, DAAP Word Count = 292. High Score Proportion = 1.0, Mean High Score = 0.08

> The walk from the church to the gravesite was long. It led through rows of tombstones, some tilted, full of cracks and moss, some illegible, some smooth and new. The air was full of the smell of boxwood, brought out by the heavy moisture. A faint smell of burning grass accompanied the muffled talk and shuffling steps of the party following the casket. There were some 30 people. A lot I thought,

> but not as many as at Vati's funeral. Mostly family. And that used to be a much bigger group. But a lot of them had died as well and then there were some that carried grudges right to this moment. How foolish. Tante Steffi did not come. Just because Anny beat her to the last spot in the grave. Anny would now rest forever with Hans, her husband. While Steffi would have to look for a spot for herself, eternally separated from Andi, Hans' brother who was buried with him. And the Gemeinde Wien was very strict there: only five people to a grave on Zentralfriedhof, that was the rule. So it was Anny, Hans, Andi and the brother's parents, Andreas and Bertha. No more. Steffi was out.
>
> The Hall where Anny's casket lay in state was full of flowers. Some on wreaths, some in vases, some just bundled. Bright colors everywhere: lime green, orange, red, white, yellow. Their smell was intense, warming the cool tiled room. All her favorite colors. The pallbearers looked professionally sad, anticipatorily working on the tip they would receive at the gravesite.
>
> When I saw her the last time she was alive, she appeared much smaller than in real life. She had lost a lot of weight. Her upper dentures were missing.

In sharp contrast to Beckett's piece, this story shows us exactly who the players are and what is going on. We are brought right into the middle of the action and the emotions. Reading the story, we feel like we are there. The piece gives a clear temporal sequence of events while providing us with the driving emotions. We are pulled into the story. This text is an example of Synthesis.

Given the very different reading experience that each piece creates, someone choosing Beckett's story as a favorite over this one would tell us a lot about his own unconscious. We could infer that he connects with feelings of alienation and emotional distance from others, or perhaps he feels estranged from some aspect of his life.

If, on the other hand, he selected as his favorite a piece like *Peripeteia* that brings him right into the action and lets him in on the character's emotions and emotional reactions, we could infer that he resonates with emotional openness. Perhaps he likes knowing his surroundings, whom he is with, and what is going on. Selecting such a piece would suggest that he likes having the warmth of human contact rather than the cool of social distance.

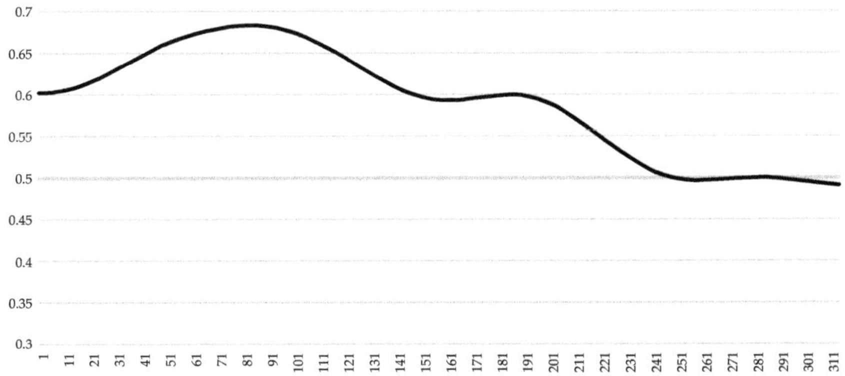

Irvin Yalom: *Three Cries*. Mean Referential Activity = 0.59, DAAP Word Count = 314, High Score Proportion = 0.79, Mean High Score = 0.12

Though I met with Helena only once many years ago, our rich hour together remains clearly etched in my mind. She was a lovely, well-spoken, forty-five year-old therapist who came to talk about her friend, Billy, and cried three times during our consultation.

Billy, who had died three months before, loomed large in her life. Their worlds had been different—he swirling in the Soho gay world, she ensconced in a fifteen year bourgeois marriage—but they had been life-long friends, meeting in the second grade and living together during their twenties in a Brooklyn commune. She was poor, he rich; she cautious, he devil-may-care; she awkward, he brimming with savoir-faire. He was blond and beautiful and taught her to drive a motorcycle and sky dive.

"Once," she reminisced with stars in her eyes, "we motorcycled for six months throughout all of South America with nothing but small packs on our back. That was the zenith of my life. Billy used to say, 'let's experience everything, let's leave no regrets, let's use up all there is and leave nothing left for death to claim.' And then, suddenly, four months ago, brain cancer and my poor Billy was dead in a few weeks."

But that was not when she cried: that happened a few minutes later.

"Last week I reached an important milestone in my life. I passed my state exams and am now a licensed clinical psychologist."

"Congratulations. That *is* a milestone."

"Milestones aren't always good."

"How so?"

"Last weekend my husband took our twelve year son and his two best friends camping and I spent much of the weekend assimilating this milestone and reviewing my life. I cleaned house, I sorted through closet after closet packed full of useless possessions, and I came upon an old forgotten album of photos of Billy that I hadn't seen for years."

This excerpt is a second example of a Synthesis text. It is by my friend and mentor, Irvin Yalom, M.D., and it shows a very polished storyteller at work. It is highly temporal—the story is clear, structured, and has causal links between events. It is also quite vivid. We can picture Helena and Billy: we see the two friends riding a motorcycle through South America, and we can feel the emotions within the story.

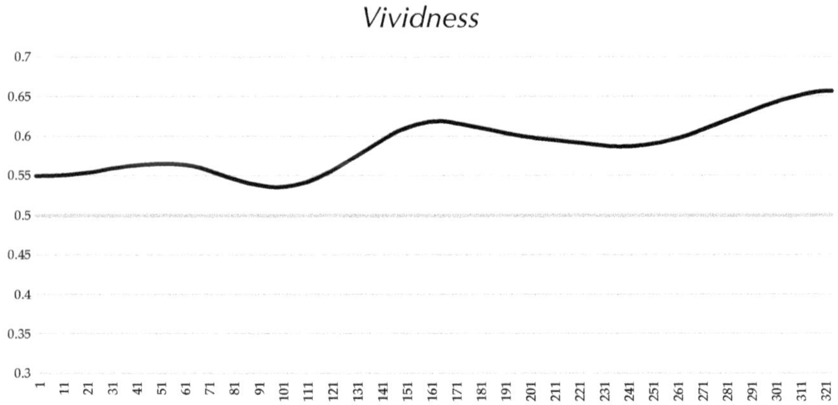

Daniel Mason: *The Piano Tuner*. Mean Referential Activity = 0.59, DAAP Word Count = 325, High Score Proportion = 1.0, Mean High Score = 0.09

In the fleeting seconds of final memory, the image that will become Burma is the sun and a woman's parasol. He has wondered which visions would remain—the Salween's coursing coffee flow after a storm, the predawn palisades of fishing nets, the glow of ground turmeric, the weep of jungle vines. For months the images trembled in the back of his eyes, at times flaming and fading away like candles, at times fighting to be seen, thrust forward like the goods of jostling bazaar merchants. Or at times simply passing, blurred freight wagons in a travelling circus, each one a story that challenged credibility, not for any fault of plot, but because Nature could not permit such a condensation of color without theft and vacuum in the remaining parts of the world. Yet above these visions, the sun rises searing, pouring

> over them like a gleaming white paint. The Bedin-saya, who interpret dreams in shaded, scented corners of the markets, told him a tale that the sun that rose in Burma was different from the sun that rose in the rest of the world. He only needed to look at the sky to know this. To see how it washed the roads, filling the cracks and shadows, destroying perspective and texture. To see how it burned, flickered, flamed, the edge of the horizon like a daguerreotype on fire, overexposed and edges curling. How it turned liquid the sky, the banyan trees, the thick air, his breath, throat, and his blood. How the mirages invaded from distant roads to twist his hands. How his skin peeled and cracked. Now this sun hangs above a dry road. Beneath it, a lone woman walks under a parasol, her thin cotton dress trembling in the breeze, her bare feet carrying her away toward the edge of perception. He watches her, how she approaches the sun, alone. He thinks of calling out to her, but he cannot speak.

This excerpt is also from a member of our Pegasus Physician Writers at Stanford group, Daniel Mason, M.D. It is taken from his first novel, which was published as a student. It is heavily poetic. The strong imagery throughout—the glow of ground turmeric, the sun washing the roads, the peeled and cracked skin—causes a high referential activity score of 0.59, with 100 percent of the line graph significantly above the 0.5 neutral line. But, we do not have a clear idea of what actually takes place in the story. There is no sequence of events or causality between the statements that gives a temporal context to the poetry. This piece is an example of Vividness.

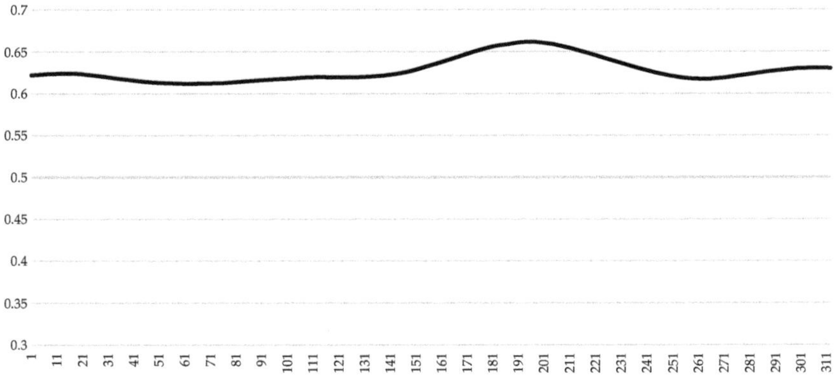

Virginia Woolf: *The Waves*. Mean Referential Activity = 0.63, DAAP Word Count = 315, High Score Proportion = 1.0, Mean High Score = 0.13

> The sun had not yet risen. The sea was indistinguishable from the sky, except that the sea was slightly creased as if a cloth had wrinkles in it. Gradually as the sky whitened a dark line lay on the horizon dividing the sea from the sky and the grey cloth became barred with thick strokes moving, one after another, beneath the surface, following each other, pursuing each other, perpetually. As they neared the shore each bar rose, heaped itself, broke and swept a thin veil of white water across the sand. The wave paused, and then drew out again, sighing like a sleeper whose breath comes and goes unconsciously. Gradually the dark bar on the horizon became clear as if the sediment in an old wine bottle has sunk and left the glass green. Behind it, too, the sky cleared as if the white sediment there had sunk, or as if the arm of a woman couched beneath the horizon had raised a lamp and flat bars of white, green and yellow spread across the sky like blades of a fan. Then she raised her lamp higher and the air seemed to become fibrous and to tear away from the green surface flickering and flaming in red and yellow fibers like the smoky fire that roars from the bonfire. Gradually, the fibers of the burning bonfire were fused into one haze, one incandescence which lifted the weight of the woolen grey sky on top of it and turned it into a million atoms of soft blue. The surface of the sea slowly became transparent and lay rippling and sparkling until the dark stripes were almost rubbed out. Slowly the arm that held the lamp raised it higher and then higher until a broad flame became visible; an arc of fire burnt on the rim of the horizon, and all round it the sea blazed gold.

This excerpt is again filled with heavily poetic language and is an example of Vividness. Virginia Woolf vividly describes the sun rising using colorful language, which is reflected in a high referential activity score of 0.63, a High Score Proportion of 1, and a Mean High Score of 0.13. However, there are no events or sequential actions that take place. She uses imagery to paint a detailed picture, but the description is not temporal—the excerpt does not tell a story. She is getting you interested, and to me she is exquisite in achieving this. She also foreshadows the plot of the book, but contains it in her metaphors in the piece.

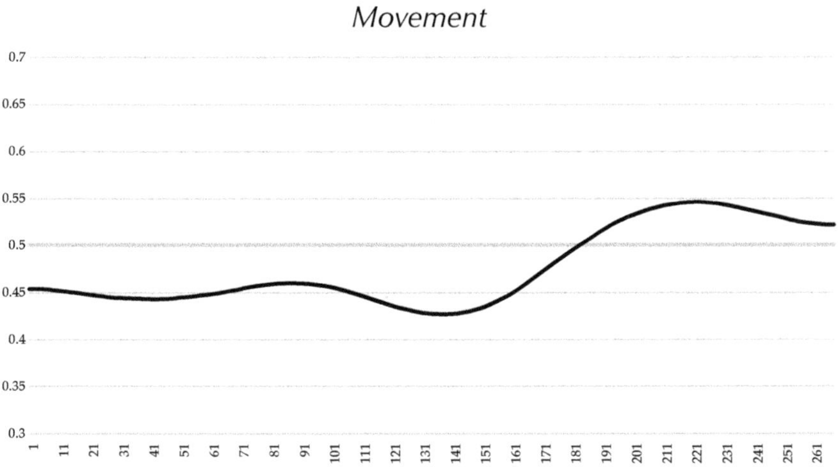

Daniel Mason: *The Second Doctor Service*. Mean Referential Activity = 0.48, DAAP Word Count = 267, High Score Proportion = 0.32, Mean High Score = 0.03

Sirs—Having read with interest Dr. Pritchard's recent report of the young woman with paroxysmal amnesia and transformation of personality, as well as Dr. Slayer's study "On the so-called Cumberland Were-wolf," I have spent the past months in deliberation over whether or not to share my own case with your readers. If I have hesitated, it is less out of concerns for privacy—pseudonyms should suffice—than the simple fact that, though bearing the title of Physician, I am but a country doctor, whose medical expertise extends little beyond those afflictions befalling the farmers and milkmaids of K—County. Indeed, I likely never would have opened your learned Journal were it not for the strange events of the past year. Most of the members of your Society, I am aware, publish with that noble aim of advancing Medicine; I write with the hope that one of them has encountered a case like my own, and so might save me before it is too late.

Unlike most illnesses, Sirs, which arise within us so insidiously, creeping through vein and fiber, unsettling our slumber, awakening within us that ineffable, horrific sense of *dis-ease*—it is possible to state the very *instant*, indeed the very Longitude and Latitude, of my affliction, being four strokes after Twelve Noon,

> on August 24, 1882, on the cusp of Mersey's Ridge outside of S—. I was returning from a sick-call. It was a warm summer day, one of those particularly golden morrows when the air is thick with motes of pollen, and the scent of rank wet grass rises from the fields.

The opening of Daniel Mason's *The Second Doctor Service* is temporal, but not very referentially active, which we see in the referential activity score of 0.48. Only 32 percent of the text is referential, and only slightly so (with a Mean High Score of 0.03). The story lays out the sequence of events—the doctor describes his motivations for writing to the journal, and then he tells the story of his disease, event by event. However, the language is not vivid or emotional. For the majority of the excerpt, we cannot picture what is happening; the author doesn't bring us into his world. There is no emotional compass to orient the events. It is only at the end when we can start to picture the scene on the warm summer day, and here the referential activity score on the graph shoots up. Given that the story is written as a letter from a doctor to a clinical journal, Mason's choice to write in a temporal but unemotional way makes sense. This is an example of Movement.

Much like Mason's *The Second Dr. Service*, the opening of *The Great Gatsby* by F. Scott Fitzgerald (Mean Referential Activity = 0.51; DAAP Word Count = 303; High Score Proportion = 0.65; Mean High Score = 0.03) is temporal, but not referential. It is another example of Movement—a kind of "play by play" writing which bypasses the emotions involved. The language doesn't transport us into the world of the author—there are no sensory details, no imagery, no emotions. But there is a story being told about why the protagonist reserves judgments, and this explanation is laid out in a temporal, sequential manner.

Now let's go through expressive writing examples from some of my patients.

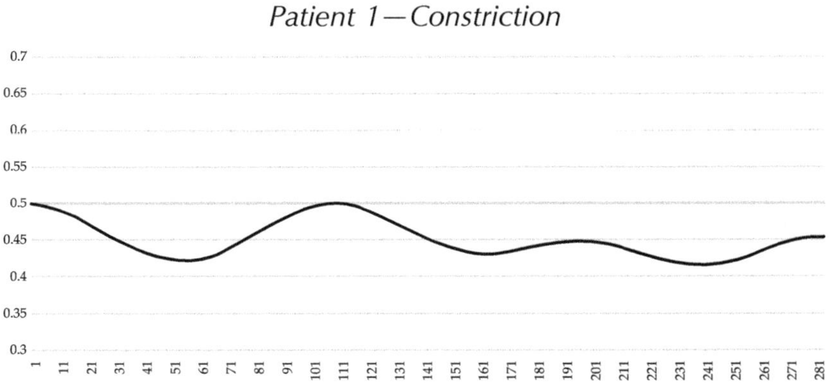

Mean Referential Activity = 0.45, DAAP Word Count = 282, High Score Proportion = 0.02, Mean High Score = 0.00

> The worst thing that has happened to me. I would have to say the worst thing, which may sound odd, would be growing up so fast. When you're young everything is simple and you are who you are. No faking to be popular and you don't think of how people want to see you. You just do and wear and say what you feel like. I miss those times when I was innocent and I feel like I had a clean start with my parents and no issues or big fights. As I got older I always have the constant struggle of being a normal teenager and then trying to please my parents. It's so hard to come home and try and be who your parents want you to be when you were just out with friends doing things that everyone does but your parents don't understand. Also I don't always have the same views as my parents on a lot of things and we don't agree which makes things difficult. Growing up has changed me and sometimes I can't even tell who I am anymore. I spend so much time in a school around people who are all a certain way and even if I don't think the same or like the same things I just have to go with it. I'm not a follower, that much I know. But a lot of the time I find myself letting people think I am and think I'm less passionate and knowledgeable than I really am. I wish I just didn't grow up and let myself succumb to the pressure and influences.

This text has low temporality and low referential activity. There is no story here. The statements do not progress in a temporal way, nor are there any causal links. There is also very little expressivity in the text, which is confirmed by a mean referential activity score of 0.45, a High Score Proportion of 0.02, and a Mean High Score of 0. The author does not link sensory or emotional experiences with expressive language. She does not bring us into her world and make us experience her story. Instead, there is a level of removal between the language and the experience she describes.

Patient 2—Synthesis

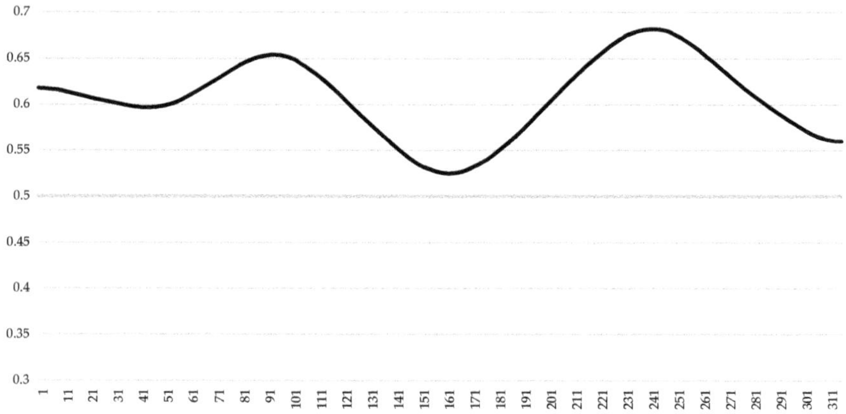

Mean Referential Activity = 0.61, DAAP Word Count = 319, High Score Proportion = 1.0, Mean High Score = 0.11

> Many years ago, I signed up to show my mare Suzy at the Horse Park on San Hill. I hadn't shown much and was pretty nervous about appearing in front of a judge. I had to ride my horse over to the show grounds, about a mile, as I didn't have a trailer. We arrived early and I found a place to tie her up while I went to the show office to pick up my number. I found out that there were seventy entries! Yikes. But I put on my penny with a big #40 on the front and back, mounted and went into the warm up arena. It was full of riders all dressed alike, all wearing the same pennies over their jackets, all wearing black helmets. I realized that I looked exactly like everyone else and that not even my age could be determined in that crowd. I could be the eight year old or the eighty year old. The realization relaxed me immediately. When my number was called, I went into the arena to ride my test knowing that I could blow it or do great

> and no one would know either way. I rode a steady test and got a big smile from the judge. I thought it was because I had a smile on my face the whole time. Since the class was so big and would go on into the afternoon, I rode home after I finished and drove back to check on the scores. Imagine my surprise to find I had come in third. Third out of seventy. I was pretty proud and at the same time knew I had been handed a great gift. Shows never bothered me after that. I knew what I was there for and what the judge or anyone else thought really didn't matter. It was just me and my horse, testing ourselves.

In contrast to Patient 1's text, this one is highly temporal and referential. The clear sequence of events delineates a story—each statement describes the next action in the narrative. It takes us by the hand and leads us through the experience, one event at a time. The mean referential activity score is high (0.61), which reflects the high level of vividness. One hundred percent of the text is above the 0.5 neutral line, and significantly so (with a Mean High Score of 0.11). The description of events is detailed—we can picture the scene and feel the nervousness, anticipation, pride, and relief. The author lets us into her world.

Patient 3—Vividness

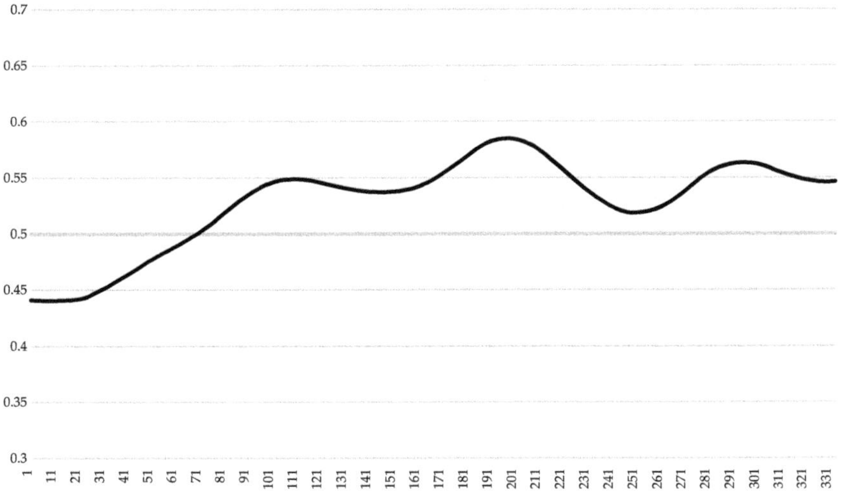

Mean Referential Activity = 0.53, DAAP Word Count = 332, High Score Proportion = 0.79, Mean High Score = 0.05

> When I daydream, it is often about owning my own stable. I understand the problems involved, labor relations, accidents, and especially the personality conflicts that inevitably arise, but in my dream facility, none of that happens. We have happy horses, happy riders, no flies, no floods, no fires. I can't think of anything happier than waking up to feed a barn full of hungry horses, all the heads poked out of the stalls calling for me to hurry. The maintenance would be ongoing but I imagine it being a kind of recreation. Kind of like building a bird house in shop class. Hard work, but fun and rewarding. I have met so many young Hispanic men at the barn where I stable my horse, and they are all hard working, caring, and quick to spot and report problems. I know we could form a great working relationship. There would have to be woods and trails, hills, too, but enough flat space for arenas. It would be great to have a vet clinic on premises like Portola Valley Training Center does. Perhaps lured there by a rent subsidy. Great idea. In addition to boarders and boarded horses, I would like to have room to house retired horses who have worked hard all their lives. Wouldn't be nice to shelter these gallant older horses and see that they have a happy old age? Maybe I'm hoping for something like that for myself and Ben. Odd though it may seem, I think a green burial business on the same site would make a nice partnership. Green burial sites usually don't allow headstones. At most the grave is marked with a plaque set into the ground. It wouldn't interfere or interrupt the running of the riding facility. And at the end of the day Ben and I would sit out in front of the barn with some of the late riders, having a beer and telling stories, maybe some tall tales.

This text is expressive, with a referential activity score of 0.53. She paints a picture and invites the reader into her daydream of owning a stable. We can picture the scene. However, we see little temporality here—there is no story, no sequential events tied together by causal links. This text has little action, only detailed imagery.

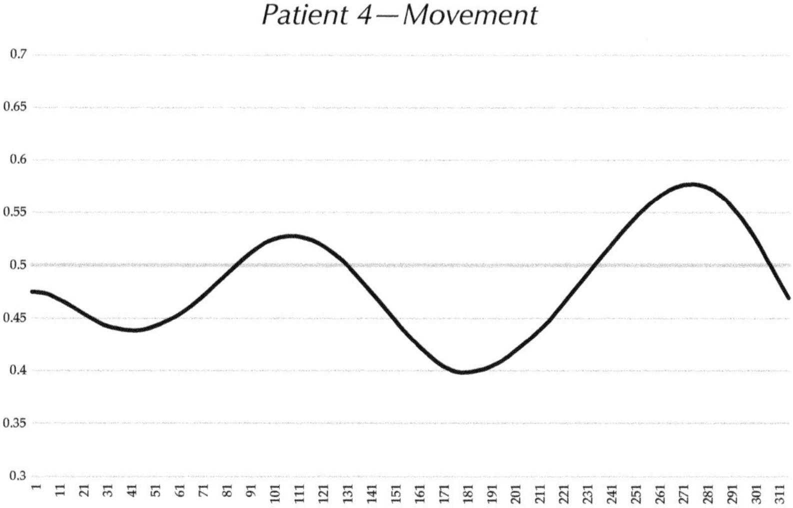

Mean Referential Activity = 0.49, DAAP Word Count = 322, High Score Proportion = 0.41, Mean High Score = 0.04

On Tuesday those kids are bothering me I'm starting to get sick of this. Wow cool bike oh I have an idea. Who can help me maybe get that bike? Maybe Eric can. Oh good I have help classes are boring can't wait till schools out. I'm hungry maybe I can go to ninos there pizza special is a good deal. Wednesday, where should he put that bike? Maybe in the church on laurel. Okay good he knows where that is. Blake wants to come that's weird I just met him and he wants to help. Maybe this will get them to stop. That is a nice looking bike better than I've had. P.E. teachers a real pain when he going to give my iPod back anyway, oh that reminds me I got to give my other to friend for his P.E. Man I hate running unless it's for a reason. Those kids won't even know what hit them. Can't wait till after school I hope Eric didn't forget. I don't care what they say I didn't steal his why can't they just learn that. Basketball was fun at lunch I'm going to do that tomorrow to. Maybe I should keep the pegs. Who doesn't put a lock on their bike wow there just asking for it to be stolen. Finally schools done okay just finish hw then get that bike. Hard to concentrate but finally done. Okay got to go find Eric where is he? Did he take the bike? Where'd he put it? Did the owner see him? Oh there he is wow he put it in the wrong place. Oh well I'll just live with this. We got to hide this better. Okay thats better now were not out in the open. Theses grips suck I'm going to take them off.

This text is temporal—the sequence of events surrounding the bike theft and resulting arrest are clearly delineated—but the referential activity is low (0.49). Only 41 percent of the text is referential, and only slightly so. Even though the text tells a story, we aren't privy to the driving emotions. We readers get the feeling that there is much more to this story than we are told. This is an adolescent boy trying to describe and explain the events leading up to him committing a crime.

These four quadrants—Constriction, Synthesis, Vividness, and Movement—correspond to the four Weinberger Adjustment Inventory (WAI) quadrants that I discussed in Chapter Three—Reactive, Suppressor, Repressor, and Non-Reactive. The Restraint axis on the WAI graph maps onto the temporal junctures axis of the expressive writing graph: Self-restraint will make it easier to package events temporally and as a story. The Distress axis on the WAI graph corresponds to the referential activity axis of the expressive writing graph: Access to emotions will facilitate the ability to express those emotions vividly.

Those with high levels of Distress but low Restraint on the WAI (Reactives) are likely to write vividly; they access their emotions easily but are less able to regulate those emotions or package them into a structured story (Vividness). Those with high Distress and high Restraint (Suppressors) may find it easier to write expressively and structure the text (Synthesis). Low levels of Distress and high levels of Restraint (Repressors) may make it easier to structure thoughts, but harder to express emotions (Movement). Finally, low Distress and low Restraint (Non-Reactives) may make both elements of the writing—expressivity and structuring a story—difficult (Constriction).

Adaptive style by distress and restraint

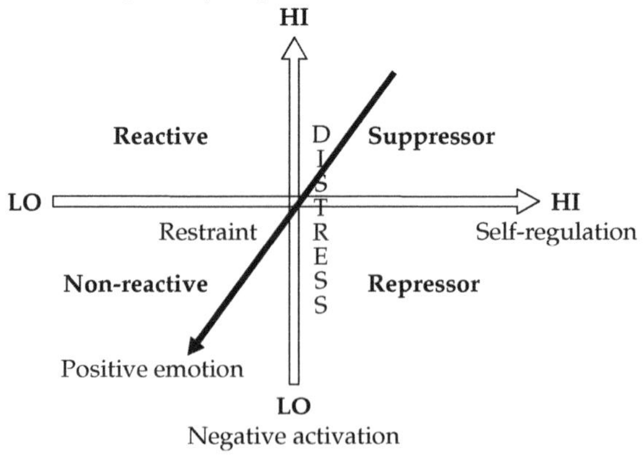

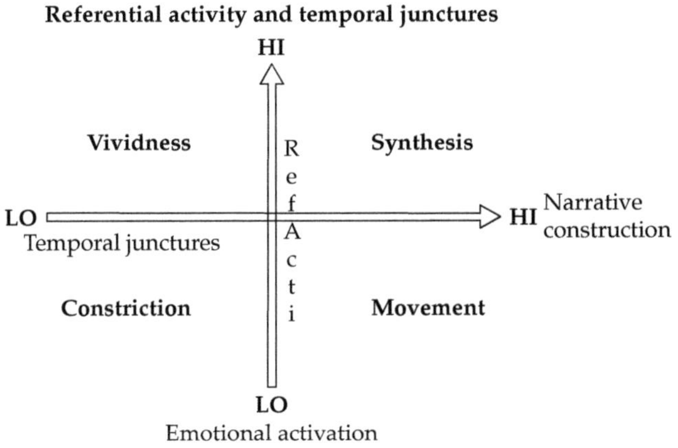

It is important to remember that these classifications are a way to simplify how to think about writing. In reality, classifying a piece is not always this clear-cut. Often we cannot so easily categorize a text into one of these four distinct types. This model can provide a framework to help us think about these concepts, but we may not find our own writings falling cleanly into one category—and that is okay, and to be expected.

I would also encourage you to use your intuition when judging your own writing. We have described how probably all humans have this innate or early nascent capacity to understand, tell, and write stories. When you have written your piece, sit back and see if you get the impression that it is a story with color. See if you feel involved or not. Then you can save yourself a great deal of all these mathematical gyrations, which appeal to only some of us with a more empirical bent.

Now, let's discuss a few expressive writing examples from students. I have removed or changed any identifying information, but have not otherwise edited the texts. I have analyzed the first 300 words of each text with the DAAP. Due to the complexity of counting temporal junctures, I recommend using word count as an indicator of temporality and will demonstrate this technique here. For the texts below I will therefore report two word counts: The "DAAP Word Count" is the number of words that were used by the DAAP program to calculate the mean referential activity score. The "Entire Text Word Count" is the total number of words that the student wrote in the allotted thirty minutes—this word count is the proxy that I use for temporality instead of temporal junctures.

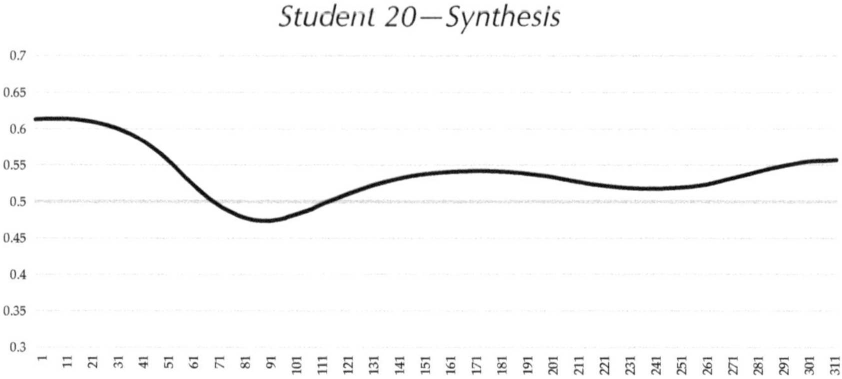

Mean Referential Activity = 0.54, DAAP Word Count = 313, Entire Text Word Count = 416, High Score Proportion = 0.86, Mean High Score = 0.05

Celebrating Christmas with my family was always something really special. Every year my grandparents, my parents, and the closest relatives gathered together on the 24th. We were used to celebrate at my grandparents' place. When they went by we started to celebrate at my parents' place. It was a real celebration because during the days of the great cold the whole family came together. However, last year I had some problems with my family and I decided not to travel home to celebrate Christmas. There were 2 reasons for that: 1) I really didn't feel to celebrate with them 2) I wanted to send a message saying don't take my presence for granted. So Christmas was coming closer and I had no flight ticket for home and I had to tell my parents why I didn't come. They were sad and I felt a bit guilty, but not that much. A few days before Christmas eve a package was delivered at my door. It was sent by my parents and it had some typical Christmas cookies and other food in it. Obviously I was happy. There was also a greeting card attached. Usually it was my mother writing such cards, but this time also my father wrote something. He wrote something like: ... so that the scent of home won't be lost, because through the webcam we can't preserve it. In the beginning I was very happy reading there words. I kept on thinking about these few words for days. I never received a message like that from my father. But as the days went by I felt a bit annoyed. At some point I figured out the thing I didn't like. I can't remember my father ever saying sweet words like these. He always was a very uncommunicative person and he never spoke

> about his feelings. The fact that he wrote these words meant that he indeed was able to do it. Therefore, the good feelings I had for his words turned in bad feelings because they came from a person I didn't know in this way. I always expected my father to be more open hearted. I am wondering why he always was so silent without expressing his feelings. In fact, when I catch up with him on the webcam he's still my old father. I always ask myself if we, my siblings and I, did enough for my parents to make them happy. To us it looks like our parents are very sad.

We begin the analysis of this piece by asking, is it a story, with a beginning, middle, and end? The beginning of a story orients us to the character and the setting. It sets the scene. We learn about the author's Christmas traditions and who is involved. Next, we look for the middle complicating action. After deciding not to join his family for Christmas, the writer receives a package from his parents with a letter from his father. The story ends as the author writes how upset he is with his father for never having expressed love or kind words before. The word count (419) is within the normal range, and there is a clear temporality within the piece—the events are told in succession and are causally linked. It is a story.

Now we look at the emotionality of the piece. Does reading this piece make you feel a particular way? How does it make you feel? How do you think the writer feels? Does the writing pull you in and make you feel these same emotions? There are some clear emotions here. The author expresses a little bit of guilt about not going home, and near the end of the piece, he writes about feeling upset, sad, and frustrated by his father. The mean referential activity is 0.54, which is within the normal range. Eighty-six percent of the text is referential, but not highly so. Some emotionality is expressed, but the author may also have some feelings that aren't entirely addressed. Because the piece is both temporally structured and emotional, we label it as Synthesis.

Now we look for any indicators of latent content lurking beneath the surface. The line graph suggests that the author backs away from some emotions. It dips significantly just before 100 words and then levels out, hovering around 0.5 for the rest of the text. What happens in the text around 100 words? Just as he switches from writing about happy times with his family to his present negative feelings, the graph drastically drops. For the remainder of the text he discusses the problems with his family, and the graph remains level, around 0.5. Although he acknowledges his emotions on the surface, the author backs away from delving deeply into how he feels or into what happened to make him feel that way.

As readers, we get the feeling that the author isn't quite telling the whole story. He mentions feeling a little bit guilty, but quickly minimizes the feeling. He refers to problems with the family and not wanting to go home for Christmas, but does not elaborate. He does not explain why he wants to send his family a message by not going home. Then, at the end of the piece, he comments that perhaps he has not done enough to make his parents happy, and that they seem very sad. This is quite a heavy statement that likely has complex emotions and a lot of history surrounding it, but he does not elaborate on any of this.

Student 20 would find it worthwhile to explore this content. Likely, he has some resistance to addressing these emotions and the difficulties with his family. Undertaking additional expressive writing tasks about this topic could elucidate how he really feels, allowing him to sort through those feelings and put them to rest.

Student 21—Constriction

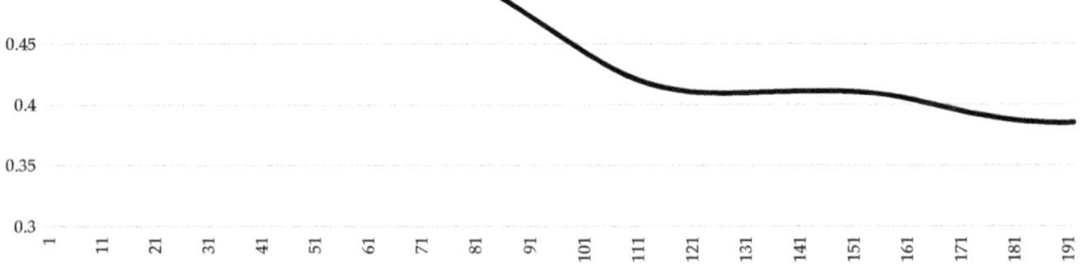

Mean Referential Activity = 0.47, DAAP Word Count = 196, Entire Text Word Count = 187, High Score Proportion = 0.42, Mean High Score = 0.05

> Writing about my experiences—or trying to do so—was a negative experience for me. In general I see myself as a very positive person,

> at least to others, but every time I was formulating my positive experience bits and pieces of negativity found its way in. I fought to keep it out and that made me unhappy to because I knew we were supposed to let go. And then, when I sat down to write about a negative experience, I couldn't think of one specific experience that I could put into words. I know there's a big cloud in my horizon that I fight hard with smiles and laughter to keep away. I know that it's filled with sadness, guilt and powerlessness. I know why the cloud is there but I can't make it go away. And I can't write about it. I don't find myself willing to push away the sun and let the storm come. It will be too big and I'm afraid I won't be able to rise again. I must wait till I know that I'm strong enough to stand against it.

This writer is a good example of someone who is very resistant to facing strong emotion through expressive writing. There is not a clear story—no true beginning, no middle, and no end. The piece is more a series of independent statements than a temporal story. She has not yet packaged a troubling event in a cohesive way; she is still processing. The word count is quite low (187), which is another indicator of resistance. The low word count also distorts the referential activity score. Generally, a word count below 300 words will not produce accurate results with the DAAP program. We must take these scores and the graph with a grain of salt.

It is clear, however, that the author does not want to approach any real emotion. There is no vivid language here; the piece does not pull us in. Although she mentions distressing emotions, she does not elaborate or give us any context. This is not a referentially active piece. With little structure and little emotion, we classify this writing as a Constriction piece.

Sometimes the task of expressive writing is a real struggle. As the author describes, we may not always write what we intended, and we may face significant emotional resistance. When confronting obstacles like these, do not be discouraged. Remember to let go and write whatever comes to mind. Over time, the process will flow more freely. Sometimes, as Student 21 experienced, we aren't ready to face distressing feelings or experiences. This often happens when we are still in the midst of a storm. But working slowly and carefully using tools like expressive writing, as we feel ready, will ultimately allow us to move beyond those emotions.

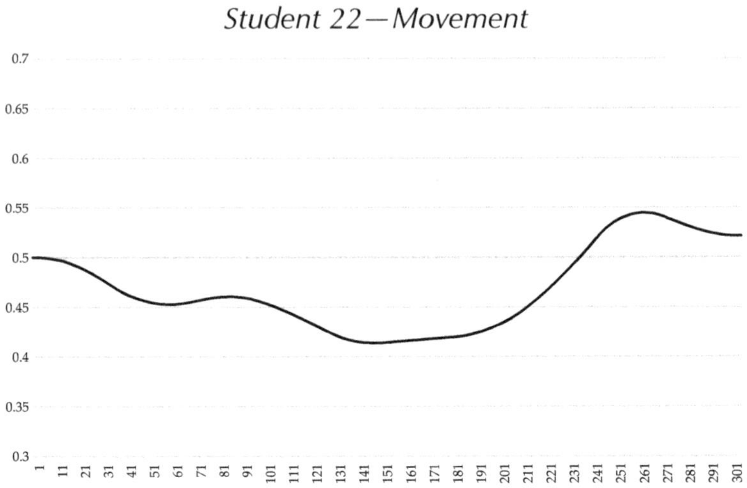

Mean Referential Activity = 0.47, DAAP Word Count = 301, Entire Text Word Count = 289, High Score Proportion = 0.23, Mean High Score = 0.03

I drop the kids and on my way home for a quick shower before heading to work. These mornings always feel like a battle. I'll first have a cereal bowl to relax a bit. I certainly deserve this quiet moment before the work day bursts in. I can read some emails in the meantime. The inbox is full and the to-do list overflowing. What should I do first? I'm still very hungry, I'll prepare a quick sandwich, nothing fancy just two pieces of bread and some Swiss cheese in between. No harm in watching a bit of Netflix while I'm eating. I'm watching another episode of the Prime Suspect. Why didn't I see it at the time? I was probably too busy then too. It is strange watching it now. It is slow but I'm still in suspense, so just half an hour longer, just one last episode. I can see that I won't do much today. The pressure is building in my stomach, like I want to throw up. But perhaps this day is not so bad. My brother would have said that I just hospitalized myself for the day. I like this thought. I don't know how it happened but I'm now watching this three-part documentary about this brilliant but self-destructive screen writer. He is so beautiful and playful in the early pictures and now so old, so fat, so broken. In tremendous honesty he deconstructs his obsessions, how he couldn't write a line without sniffing a line, how he couldn't escape the curse of the males in his family, how he neglected his children. When telling how he cried all the way back

> from his weekly meeting with his abandoned child, I find myself crying too.

This text is somewhat temporal—A leads to B, which leads to C—although many causal links between events are missing. It has a beginning, middle, and end, but it leaves us with many unanswered questions: Where does he drop the kids off? Why do these mornings feel like a battle? Why does the author feel so pressured? Why does he cry at the end? The word count, significantly lower than average, indicates some resistance. We can classify it as a story, although the author must do some additional processing in order to package these thoughts into a clear narration.

The mean referential activity is 0.47, significantly below the average. The High Score Proportion and Mean High Score values are also low. At face value, the text seems to express emotionality; the author feels overwhelmed, anxious, and sad. However, he does not dig deeply into any of these emotions. While acknowledging his unhappiness, he backs away from exploring its cause and what it really feels like, which is reflected in the low referential activity score. This writing is an example of a Movement text.

The graph dips particularly low between 100 and 200 words. At this point in the text, the author backs way off his feelings of distress and suggests that the day may not be so bad after all. The dip in referential activity here suggests that this optimism is an attempt to hide deeper, more upsetting emotions.

The graph then peaks between 200 and 300 words, which corresponds to the author's description of the documentary character. Student 22's writing gets significantly more expressive and vivid when describing another's sorrows, rather than his own. There is something in the documentary character's plight that Student 22 identifies with. By displacing his emotions onto a proxy, he can symbolically express them, which protects his conscious mind from having to face his own feelings.

The text is highly metaphoric, which gives us hints about the underlying emotion and latent content. Phrases like "these mornings always feel like a battle," "the work day bursts in," and "the to-do list overflowing" create a feeling of tension. The metaphor here is one of battle and fighting. The author perhaps feels pulled in too many directions, overwhelmed, and constantly battling how to both meet his work obligations and spend time with his children. He seems to feel unable to keep up. He could benefit from exploring this topic more deeply and focusing on these emotions in future expressive writing exercises. Over time, he may find himself molding these thoughts and feelings into a more structured story, with causal links and temporal sequencing, and become more able to fully express his emotions. This writing process could significantly help him to work through these difficult emotions, rather than feeling stuck in them and overwhelmed.

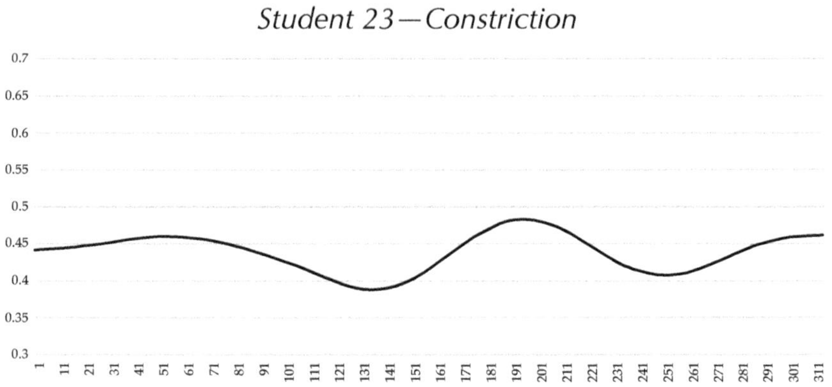

Mean Referential Activity = 0.44, DAAP Word Count = 316, Entire Text Word Count = 521, High Score Proportion = 0.0, Mean High Score = 0.0

> Is this glowing letter of recommendation really about me? I'm numb. Maybe all that "self pride stinks" mantra from the family has numbed me to being able to see praise about myself. Hmm Thanks, Gram. Its amazing to be called bright and motivated and a joy to have in class. How about that? I'm a joy. I know part of it is not feeling smart because of the math struggles. And the ridicule of Sister Helen and others that I couldn't find my way out of a paper bag. Why would a teacher do that? I think I'll take this letter writers word over those nay sayers. I'd rather be a joy than looked on as stupid. I'm amazed how that negativity still hides in me. The maybe I'm not good enough mantra. I should post this letter where I can see it every day as an antidote to the mean teachers. I Do work hard. I Do study hard. I Do try for scholarly work. It's the warring forces of the nay sayers and my cheerleaders. I have to decide who I want to let win this tug of war. Every time I do well in a class a little voice inside goes Yes! Take that people who didn't believe in me!

> How do I get past them? How do I stop letting them have this much power? Stuff like this. Psychological talk back. I like that. I don't want to be a victim. I learn differently sometimes but different isn't bad. It's different. Plain and simple. Like me—shoot straight, work hard and be called a joy in class. I can live with that. Why is learning so important to me? I think because it takes me to other worlds but also in the opposite direction and helps me learn about me. The inside me. It feels good. Like a most satisfying journey. Love library reading rooms. Love the first day of a new class. Love the triumph of the final dot on a completed term paper. Its all there for me. Sister Helen, don't try to take that away from me! Wonder if she's still alive? Wrecking havoc and pain on yet another generation. Hope not. What painful place is she coming from to feel compulsed (is that a word?) to do this to students? That helps me hate her a little less. But only a little. Maybe it's a good lesson for me. To heed how I treat my own students. That's a gift that can come from this. Kind of. Back to the letter. Can I frame it? Can I mail a copy to Sister Helen? Ha. That would be fun. Best of all, I think is to move forward. This letter writer knows me now and celebrates me. This is a gift to me and a stronger voice then the negative. I need to start hearing it. I want to start hearing it. How long do I want to be a victim? Expiration date on that long overdue. Think I will post it in my home and in my heart. After all, I'm a joy!

Though the word count is within the normal range, we do not see a clear progression of events here, or a beginning, middle, and end. With a High Score Proportion of 0, the DAAP curve stays in the unreferential activity zone (i.e., the curve stays below 0.5), and the mean referential activity score is 0.44, an indication of low vividness or emotionality. Again, this writing is an example of Constriction.

This text was written in response to the prompt, "Write about a positive event," but there is a noticeable lack of positive emotionality. We are left with the question: When writing about such a happy event, what stops the author from writing with vivid, positive emotions? What is she holding back? Perhaps the author is backing away from a deeper layer of emotion.

She does begin to express happiness just before word 350, when she describes everything that she loves about school. The remainder of the text is infused with a lot of self-critical, negative memories and emotions. This is another example of how we don't always write about what we consciously intend to write about. Often, hints at what we are repressing, or what needs to be processed, creep into the writing, even when we deliberately try to write about a happy experience.

This is the deeper, latent content that the author is resisting. Her memories of Sister Helen and the associated anxiety would be a good place for Student 23 to focus on when following up with future expressive writings. Because they have not been processed, these thoughts and feelings seep into even her most positive life events. Expressive writing can help her to structure the memories, digest them, and free herself from these distressing emotions.

Student 24—Synthesis

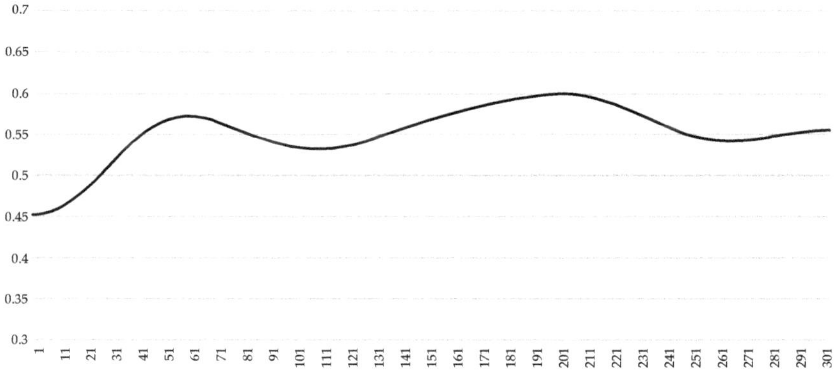

Mean Referential Activity = 0.55, DAAP Word Count = 302, Entire Text Word Count = 529, High Score Proportion = 0.91, Mean High Score = 0.06

> This week I ended a friendship. Well, I'm not sure that *I* ended it, or if my friend and I ended it mutually. Either way, the experience was sad and uncomfortable. I'd met this person in 2010 when my then-boyfriend and I were still newly dating. This woman, we'll call her T., was dating a friend of my boyfriend, but her own relationship was in flux, possibly on the verge of breaking up. She started blogging about her situation, and I supported her writing. We got to know each other initially, as many people do these days, through online venues—blogs and Facebook—before actually meeting in person. But by the time we met, it felt as though we were becoming friends already. During the course of the next two years, we would

> exchange numerous emails—often in which she approached me for support and advice as her relationship ended and she struggled with that situation. She was also having financial difficulty but wanted to start a new business that would use her writing skills in a social media venue. Our friendship continued both through email (as she lived in Oregon most of the time) and in person whenever possible. We saw each other at local music events, met for coffee, and so on. I supported her work, and she supported mine. We talked about shoes and men and life. However, after my boyfriend and I broke up at the end of 2011, it seemed that the contact T. and I had became limited to Facebook. I tried numerous times to get together with her, and yet she put me off with "too busy" and "not enough time." I sent her emails asking for advice (as she had with me two years earlier) that went unanswered for weeks. By this time she was in a new relationship, had gotten her blog and social media page off the ground (with much success), and taken on a day job to ease her financial issues. In short, her life had come together, but she had "no time" for our friendship, except to exchange comments on Facebook pages. I, on the other hand, missed seeing her in person and was moving away from social media as a way to make and maintain friendships. The novelty of Facebook had worn off for me (as it has for most of my long-time friends), and personal interaction in "the real world" was my priority. As much as I wanted to maintain a friendship with her, it felt as though things were on her terms only—and those terms were Facebook friends or nothing. Which, to me, is not a friendship at all; it's a voyeuristic experience. And, in fact, she did confirm that those were her "terms" in the email exchange that brought our three-year friendship to a close. It saddens me to think that her part in our friendship was, perhaps, based mostly on her needs at the time. And to realize that she really has pulled away from me since the end of my previous romantic relationship. She continues to maintain a friendship (again, mostly online as far as I know) with my ex-boyfriend.

The word count is within the normal range, and the text has a clear temporal sequence of events, with a beginning, middle, and end. The author sets the scene with background information about the relevant players, and then leads us through the events of the breakup with her friend, sequentially and in detail. This is a story.

The mean referential activity is 0.55, which is within the normal range. With a High Score Proportion of 0.91, the curve stays above 0.5 for the majority of the text, indicating that the author is emotionally connected to what she is writing. Rather than backing away or repressing her feelings, she gets into the heart of the matter. She allows herself to fully feel and express her emotions, and she has processed the event enough to be able to package them into a cohesive story. This is a Synthesis text.

With practice, and by utilizing tools like the DAAP program, your expressive writing style may evolve over time. You might find that you begin to naturally produce more Synthesis texts as your writing becomes more temporal and more referential, particularly if you revisit the same topic or experience repeatedly. Writing in this way not only helps you process your life experiences, but it can aid in your process of self-discovery. There are often clues about your unconscious mind hidden between the lines on the page. By learning how to recognize and decipher these clues, you can become adept at interpreting your writing in a way that gives you insight into your unconscious mind and ultimately improves your life.

Your expressive writings are generated by you and accessible to your empirical or hermeneutic analysis. In the next chapter (Chapter Seven), we will discuss how to analyze dreams and give you a model for how to approach your writings hermeneutically. We usually have to do this with dreams because—honestly—they are simply too complex to yield to empirical investigation of the type that we have described here. But over the many years of teaching this class, I have been ever so impressed with how many people can approach texts hermeneutically, and once again gain privileged access to their secret mind.

CHAPTER SEVEN

The royal road to the unconscious: dream analysis

When do dreams tell you something about yourself?

As humanity has known for thousands of years, our demons often come to visit at night, while we are sleeping. Across cultures, throughout history, and despite all of our waking life differences, once we lay our heads to rest each night human beings are united by one common experience—dreaming. We all know what it is like to close our eyes and be flooded with fantastical stories and movie-like imagery. Our dream life can be rich and vast, but what does it all mean? Some, like the ancient Greeks, believe that dreams have a prophetic quality. Others have experienced moments of great insight when fast asleep, like Albert Einstein's Theory of Relativity or James Watson with the solution to the genetic puzzle. Many of us emerge each morning with a sense that there is a message hidden within our dreaming minds.

On average, each of us will spend one third of our lifetime asleep. And we are not alone in our need to slumber—all animals sleep. The question is, why? As Dr. Allan Rechtschaffen (1971) said, "If sleep does not serve an absolutely vital function, then it is the biggest mistake the evolutionary process ever made." Despite how much time we spend nestled in bed, we do not yet conclusively know the function of sleep or dreaming.

It has been so challenging to solve these mysteries in part because dreams are inherently problematic to scientifically study. After all, how do we psychologically investigate a phenomenon that by definition occurs only when the subject is unconscious? However, the unconscious nature of dreaming is precisely what makes it so interesting. In art analysis (Chapter Five) and expressive writing (Chapter Six), we consciously steer our efforts to access the unconscious. We use clues found in our waking life to unearth deep feelings and thoughts. In dream analysis, the object of inspection—the dream—is a direct creation of the unconscious. The only conscious element of the process is the recall, allowing for a more pure glimpse into the unconscious.

Because the unconscious element of dreaming limits the range of methods for data collection, many of the psychological theories on dreaming are founded in practice-based evidence, which is the real life experience of observing and talking with patients over an extended period of time. The theories that have emerged are diverse and contradictory, from Sigmund Freud's assertion that dreams reveal our deepest selves to Crick's hypothesis that we "dream in order to forget" as a mental self-cleansing mechanism (Crick & Mitchison, 1983).

Freud first popularized the idea that dreams are a reflection of unconscious processes, calling dreams "the royal road to the unconscious." He theorized that dreams are a symbolic, highly condensed language and act as metaphors for wish fulfillments, often sexual in nature. Freud argued that because the content of the unconscious tends to be disturbing or forbidden, our minds disguise these wish fulfillments, which can be repressed desires, emotions, thoughts, or unresolved conflicts, by using symbols and metaphors. His way of coming to this conclusion was based purely on clinical data from the psychoanalysis of his patients. He summarized this work in his seminal *The Interpretation of Dreams* (1900a), which is still available today. But as important as this book was in my life, I also now know that his basic theory was flawed and curiously reductionist. As we will see, with modern investigations of neuroscience, we will arrive at different theories and conclusions, none of them definitive, but most of them promising to move the field forward.

To begin with, in 1953, researchers Eugene Aserinsky and Nathaniel Kleitman discovered that dreaming occurred most often when subjects were in Rapid Eye Movement (REM) sleep. When subjects are awakened during REM sleep, they typically report elaborate, vivid, emotional dreams. In the 1960s, Michel Jouvet's research demonstrated that the pontine brain stem, a very deep brain structure, is a critical player in REM sleep (Jouvet & Jouvet, 1963).

In 1977, J. Allan Hobson took a stand against Freud's "royal road to the unconscious" theory by presenting a theory entitled "activation-synthesis" with his colleague Robert McCarley. Hobson and McCarley argued that dreaming is merely a product of random neuronal bursts in the brain that originate in the pontine brain stem and bounce around the cortex during REM sleep. According to Hobson and McCarley, analyzing a dream for psychological meaning has little value, as there is no deeper significance. Rather than the products of unconscious thoughts and emotions, dreams occur as the brain tries to make sense of the nonsensical input from the pontine brain stem. As much as these findings seemed to deal a deathblow to any dream theory that postulated that these nightly events have meaning, clinicians were very reluctant to give up this way of exploring patients' problems.

The meaning of dreams was resurrected when Dr. David Foulkes (1962) demonstrated that the Non-Rapid Eye Movement (NREM) sleep state also contains dreams. Subjects awakening from NREM sleep report dreams that are more concise, thought-like, and less bizarre than REM dreams. However, it is difficult to determine if these dreams actually occurred during a NREM cycle, or if the subject remembered a dream that occurred earlier in the night during a REM period.

Mark Solms (1995) further challenged Hobson and McCarley's theory with the discovery that the pontine brain stem is not the only brain structure responsible for dreaming: if the pontine brain stem is damaged, dreams persist. Thus, dreaming may be more than just random firings from the brain stem. He also showed with clinical studies that the persisting dreams had more NREM characteristics. So, we seem to have two types of dreams: REM, which are bizarre and generally tend to occur soon after we go to sleep in the early parts of the night; and NREM dreams, which happen as the night comes to an end (Suzuki et al., 2004). These little concise tales are worthy of clinical attention and seem to carry meaning in a way that REM dreams do not.

As scientific technology improved, we learned more about the neuroscience related to sleep. Throughout the night, our brains phase in and out of REM and NREM sleep in ninety minute alternating cycles, entering the first REM cycle about one and a half hours after falling asleep. As the night progresses, the REM phases become longer and longer. NREM sleep is further divided into three substages, of which stage 1 is the lightest and stage 3 is the deepest. Each stage has distinct brain waves, chemical processes, and active areas of the brain. Due to the cycles of REM and NREM sleep, NREM dreams typically occur upon falling asleep and upon awakening (Oudiette et al., 2012). Interestingly, the brain structures involved in dreaming are similar to those involved in emotional activation, that is, the limbic system as discussed in Chapter Two.

Lucid dreaming occurs when we know that we are dreaming. Some believe that in this state the dreamer can control her actions, the characters, or the environment in the dream and thus arrive at useful solutions to conflicts and dilemmas. The science backing up these claims is not very solid, but the idea remains alive and well, and sometimes even reaches mystical proportions. For a very good erudite discussion of this phenomenon, along with a good explication of efforts to create a taxonomy of dreams, please refer to John Crowley's 2015 article in *Harper's Magazine*. There is a more recent finding in dream research that shows that as we prepare to go to sleep, we can "seed" our dreaming by thinking about a problem intensely, maybe making a list about it or reading about it (Solms & Turnbull, 2002). Then, we dream about it. I commonly experience this seeding phenomenon, as do my patients—and sometimes it even leads to new insights and solutions. However, the ability to control dreams has not been proven. Personally, even when I seed the subject matter of a dream, I never have the feeling of steering the dream material in any significant way. The dream emerges in all its poetic beauty.

In another important sense it is true that we are responsible for our dream content. We will discuss this in more detail below in our sections on how to approach the analysis of dreams. In my clinical work, I assume that the dreamer is the "director" of his dream—the person that places experiences and symbols together in a highly personalized way. To make a dream useful to yourself, you should embrace this assumption. Then your dream can lead you to the hidden parts of your mind. We will examine more about this when we discuss the work of George Lakoff below.

As the field continued to evolve, researchers began to debate the role of dreams in memory processing. Robert Stickgold published a paper in 2003 with Hobson and colleagues, arguing that sleep does not play a role in the consolidation of episodic, emotional memories (Fosse, Fosse,

Hobson, & Stickgold, 2003). However, researcher Jie Zhang challenged this with his paper in 2005, which proposed a theory that dreams are a product of transferring information from temporary storage to permanent storage. Zhang suggests that REM dreams represent the transfer of procedural memories, such as remembering how to perform a skill, while NREM dreams process and encode emotionally charged, episodic memories (personal events), like the birth of a child.

When this transfer contains information that is difficult to live with or to explain, the unconscious taps us on the shoulder by producing an emotional narrative and asks, where should this information be stored? The emotional, psychologically relevant dreams are a product of our minds deciding where to file the information, or in its extreme form, awaken us with a nightmare when the brain cannot see how to transfer a particularly difficult and even traumatic piece of information from our working memory space into permanent memory.

According to this idea, the dream itself is inherently meaningful. Our minds produce the scenes and stories in their entireties, and if we can remember and decode the imagery, we can learn about our unconscious mind. The other possibility is that the more meaningful element of dream analysis is the process of consciously recollecting and piecing together the dream. In this model, the brain produces the imagery (or fragments of imagery) without any deeper meaning, and upon awakening, we reflect and turn the imagery into a story that has personal significance. It is the way that we interpret, remember, and reconstruct the dream, rather than the dream itself, that reflects our deep emotions, thoughts, and memories.

Hobson came around to the idea that dreams may have meaning, publishing a paper in 2009 which theorized that REM sleep may act as a virtual model of the world. In 2010, Stickgold then hypothesized that dreaming serves an adaptive role much like that of the default network during our waking state (Wamsley & Stickgold, 2010). When our brains are "at rest," the default network (discussed in Chapter Two) is activated to process the past and plan for the future (Stickgold & Ellenbogen, 2008). According to Stickgold, when we sleep our minds continue to process and plan by piecing together different memory fragments. Our dreams act as a virtual model of waking life.

More and more evidence suggests that one function of sleep is memory consolidation. Sleeping after learning a task improves the performance of that task, and NREM sleep and dreaming appears to be particularly involved in memory formation. Studies have also shown that sleep preferentially improves personal, emotional memories.

Still, the debate on the purpose of sleep continues: in 2011 Jerome Siegel published a paper stating that sleep's primary function is to conserve energy and regulate behavior. He argued that the role of REM sleep is still a mystery, especially given that there have not been any memory, health, or overall cognitive impairments associated with the suppression of REM sleep in humans. However, lethal effects have been reported in studies of rats that are deprived of REM or NREM sleep.

Ultimately, the debate on sleep and dreams is likely to be ongoing, with opinions going back and forth with the ebb and flow of scientific advancements. That said, I believe that learning the language of dreams can expose hidden aspects of our minds. The trick is in understanding which dreams contain elements of the unconscious, and which are simply products of nonsensical brain activity. As I discussed in Chapter One, there are three different types of mental activity: conscious, unconscious, and nonconscious. Unconscious processes are normally outside of our awareness but, with effort, can be brought into our consciousness. These are the processes that the techniques in this book focus on. Nonconscious mental activity is comprised of neuronal processes that are never accessible to our conscious awareness, like the random discharges of neurons from the pontine brain stem, as Hobson and McCarley found. Some dreams may reflect unconscious mental activity and give insight into deep thoughts and emotions, while others may be products of nonconscious processes that do not contain any psychological meaning. In this chapter I will discuss how to distinguish between meaningful and meaningless dreams, as well as how to record dreams efficiently and analyze those that are psychologically significant (Hill & Knox, 2010).

We do not always remember our dreams exactly the way they occurred, and often over time the memory of a dream will change and shorten, particularly if it contains repressed emotions or information that is difficult to face. Editing out the darker elements of a memory or dream is called motivated forgetting. Take the example of "The War of Ghosts," which researcher Matthew Hugh Erdelyi used to test the ability of a nine-and–a-half-year-old girl, Karina, to recall a story accurately.

The story told to Karina was about two Native Americans who were approached by five warriors in a canoe. The warriors explained that they were going to war and invited the two Native Americans to go with them. One of the Native Americans refused to go, saying that he could be killed and his family would worry, while the other went with the warriors. The six men then went up the river where they fought, and many were killed. Then one of the warriors said that the Native American was hit, and the Native American thought, "They must be ghosts." The Native American did not feel any pain. He returned home and told his family that he had fought in a war with ghosts. Then the sun rose, and he collapsed. Black liquid spilled from his mouth, and he was dead.

After hearing the story twice, Karina first recited the story as follows:

> One day two young men went down to the river to hunt for seals. Suddenly they heard war cries. They heard the sound of paddles splashing in the water. The young men thought this was a war party and hid themselves behind a log. Soon they saw a canoe coming towards them. There were five Indians in the canoe. One of them asked the young men "What do you think? Will you join us? We are going to war on the people." One of the young men said, "I have no arrows"! The Indian replied "we have arrows in the canoe." Then one of the young men said, "I cannot go for my family does not know where I am; but you can go." Soon they departed, one to war and one to his family. They soon arrived at a village further south than Kalama. The villagers soon came to the waterfront and started a battle. Many people from both sides died. Soon the young man heard an Indian warrior say, "We better leave, that man got hit." So they left for Egulac. The young man then went home and lit a fire and told his story. When he was done he sat there to sunrise and then fell down. Something black came out of his mouth. His face was twisted. He was dead.

Some nine months later, Karina's attempt to recall the story had changed to this:

> One day two peasant farmers went fishing in a swamp. They had caught a couple of fish. Then suddenly an Indian war canoe came. The two men hid behind an old rotting moldy log. The chief knowing people were there asked if anyone wanted to join his tribe. One of the men was about to say yes but his friend persuaded him not to by telling him how heartbroken his wife and children would be if he joined the tribe. The friend told the family and told them not to mention the incident again to him, so they never did

and they lived happily ever after and never mentioned the incident to him scared he might actually leave them and they would all be heartbroken.They all lived happily ever after. The End.

Over time, Karina not only forgets a substantial amount of the story, but she omits very specific elements of the story—the scary parts. There is no fighting, no black substance dribbling from the man's mouth, and no death. Karina now ends the story "happily ever after" with both men at home with their families, rather than going off to war. She cleaned it up, eliminating the negative elements and reshaping the story. All of the unpleasant events in the story have been purged from her memory. She has also packaged the story into a more concise narrative. The story shortens from 327 words to 224 words in the initial recall, and eventually to 133 words in the final recall. She did not do that consciously and deliberately. Rather, she unconsciously molded the story to fit her preexisting concept of reality—that life should be happy, not scary.

This case study of Karina could also have been used in our previous chapter on narration, storytelling, and expressive writing, as the material generated by us when we write or tell a story is sometimes subject to the same types of distortions that we observe taking place in Karina's stories. We chose to place it here because we wanted to make the important point about dream narrations not necessarily being exact transcriptions. Despite this fact, dreams are often still clinically useful.

Another point of emphasis is that Freud's idea that dreaming codes and disguises because of latent sexual content is, as I said before, too reductionist and does not fit with what we have come to expect dreams to represent. Instead, there are disguises for many other themes in our dreams that clearly are not of a sexual nature: dreaming of death, departure, grief, terror, threat, and illness, for instance. These themes are not easily shoehorned into a sexual framework. As Wittgenstein said, in order to learn from Freud, you have to be very critical.

Much like how Karina alters "The War of Ghosts," we, too, are apt to shorten, simplify, and distort our dreams upon recalling them. Over time, the discrepancies between the actual dream and our reconstructed version of it become even more pronounced. In order to get the most accurate representation possible of your dreams, I recommend you keep a pen and paper by the bed and write your dreams down immediately upon awakening. You could also keep a voice recorder next to your bed and narrate the dream rather than writing it down. These techniques will minimize the opportunity for forgetting, altering, or reconstructing the dream. If you have difficulty remembering your dreams, don't give up. The process usually becomes easier over time, and you will likely be able to remember more and more of your dreams as you continue to record them.

Now let's discuss how to analyze our own dreams and determine which are meaningful, and which should be discarded. As Hobson theorized, some dreams are likely products of random neuronal discharges that produce images and have little, if any, psychological meaning. We might remember these dreams, but because of their nonsensical and chaotic nature, we may have difficulty piecing a story together. They can feel very emotional but still lack meaning. Dreams that are less complicated, less chaotic, and more story-like are more likely to have psychological relevance.

Nightmares are a phenomenon that we are all familiar with. Many of us have experienced the fear of being chased or harmed in our dreaming life. These are a distinct class of dream that often occurs around 3 am. They represent traces of emotionally charged memory that were formed under traumatic circumstances. In essence, the brain is replaying a traumatic event that it has not put to rest. Our minds have difficulty processing the event or moving past it, causing the trauma to pop up in the form of a nightmare. The highly emotional foundation of these dreams can make them very difficult to eradicate.

The first step in analyzing a dream is to determine whether or not it is a story. Does it have a beginning, a middle complicating action, and a conclusion? Or is it a jumble of random and incongruent scenes and pieces of information? Sometimes when we dream, it is just that—a random discharge of information and memories. If the dream falls into this category, we discard it as psychologically meaningless. However, if the dream tells a cohesive story, it may have some meaning.

Usually the beginning of the story serves to orient the characters and scenario, the middle presents some kind of complicating action, and the end acts as a summation. The events are typically told in a chronological order: Humpty dumpty sat on a wall (the beginning orientation), then he had a great fall (the middle complication action), then he couldn't be put back together again (the end summation). If these three sections are present and they are told in a logical order, we conclude that the dream is a story.

In the second step, we look at the emotionality of the dream. Does the story have a clear emotional tone, or is it flat? If there are strong emotions throughout the dream, it is another indicator that it contains psychological meaning.

Often an event from our waking hours primes a dream. The related elements we see in the dream are called the day residue. When we spend the day at the beach, we may have an ocean related dream; if we catch up with an old friend, he may pop up in our dreams later that night. Day residue is a third indicator, in addition to structure and emotionality, that a dream has meaning and is motivated by unconscious processes.

Next, we look for the metaphor within the dream. Metaphors are linguistic devices that link two normally unrelated objects or actions in order to express an idea, usually phrased as "A is B." The metaphor, "love is a journey," equates two literally unrelated concepts—love and a journey—in order to express the idea that love is a process that evolves and changes over time.

Psychologically meaningful dreams tend to be highly symbolic and metaphoric—the images, characters, and events often represent something other than what they appear to be in the dream. George Lakoff, a cognitive linguist, argues that we use metaphors to explain complex and abstract ideas in terms that are more concrete. Not only do we do this in our waking life, but also in our dream life. These metaphors are then broken down into sub-metaphors, which are used to create the dream imagery. If the metaphor is "love is a journey," the dream imagery may involve a train ride or a bridge, for example.

Lakoff (1993) suggests that our unconscious mind structures dreams with overarching metaphors that are chosen from a pool of conceptual metaphors. We each have a distinct pool of metaphors, depending on our personal experiences and memories. For example, an airplane pilot is likely to use travel as a metaphor. By orchestrating the metaphorical imagery, the unconscious acts as the stage director of the dream (either while we are asleep, or when we consciously remember the dream and piece it together). Our unconscious uses these metaphors to express concerns, thoughts, or emotions that our conscious mind may be resisting. By disguising the literal expression of these ideas, they can be more safely and delicately expressed. Thus, we may not be immediately, consciously aware of the true meaning of our dreams. Understanding the metaphor, particularly in the context of our life, is the key to decoding the meaning of a dream.

Lakoff argues that there are two primary interpretations of a dream—that of an external interpreter and that of the dreamer himself. The former is the weaker of the two, as an external interpreter cannot fully understand the meaning of a dream without knowing the context of the dreamer's life. The dreamer, on the other hand, can ultimately judge what meaning certain imagery or metaphors have within her life.

We can usually categorize the dream metaphors into a handful of grand themes: birth, growing up, relationships, achievement, love, sickness, separation, loss, and death. More than one of these themes can be present in a single dream.

The final element of dream analysis is to accept that each of us is the director of our own dreams. Our life experiences lend shape to the characters, sequence of events, and the outcome. So, even when a dream may seem unpleasant, frightening, or confusing, some part of us was motivated to depict or remember the events in that way. Teasing out that motivation can give us insight into even more hidden aspects of our emotions and thinking. Students 15, 16, 17, and 18 below are good examples of this concept.

If a dream is a clear story, contains vivid emotions, has day residue, is structured according to a metaphor, and can be categorized into one of the grand themes, the chances are good that it is worth paying attention to. We must remember that even meaningful dreams can have many valid interpretations, and that, ultimately, it is up to the dreamer to decide what meaning his dream holds. In this way, a dream is like a song or poem. We cannot forget that we are the authors of our own dreams.

Let's take a look at one of my recurring dreams. Whenever I am feeling overwhelmed or overworked, I dream that I am in some kind of transit station—an airport, a bus station, or a train station, for example. I am overloaded with luggage with suitcases in each hand and a backpack. As I hurry to catch my flight or bus, all kinds of obstacles start to appear. The wheels fall off my suitcase and signs point in the wrong direction. As I become increasingly aware of the fact that I am going to miss the flight, bus, or train, I start to feel a heavy feeling of panic. The more panicked I become, the more ridiculous the obstacles get. Suddenly a balance beam appears with water underneath that I have to cross. Then I have to traverse an icy sidewalk. No matter how hard I try, I can't keep up, and I miss whatever mode of transit I was rushing to make.

We first need to determine whether my dream is a story or not. The scene is set in the airport with my luggage, the series of obstacles presents the complicating action, and the dream concludes when I miss my flight. With all three necessary elements present, we conclude that it is a story.

We now assess the emotionality of the dream. Is a vivid emotion driving the dream? Is it emotionally charged? There is a clear, strong sense of panic, fear, frustration, and anger. No matter how hard I try, I know that I am not going to make the flight. The emotionality is my second indicator that this is a meaningful dream.

Now, we look at the metaphor in the dream to determine what it says about my unconscious emotions and thoughts. The metaphor is clearly travel, but a clue as to what this stands for lies in the recent events of my life that have led up to the dream. This dream usually occurs when I am feeling overwhelmed with work obligations that I feel panicked about completing. Typically, I have just returned from a trip to Europe, and I know that I am going to be swamped with emails, duties, and people who need something from me. Travel is acting as a metaphor for success. Just as I do in the dream, I worry in my real life that, no matter how hard I try, I will not be able to keep up. The grand theme here is achievement. Given that I have usually just returned from a trip when I have this dream, the travel theme is also a clear day residue.

Let's go through this process again with a second dream of mine. While Freud's wish fulfillment theory is sometimes true, dreaming is not always quite that simple. As I see in clinical practice, not all dreams are wish fulfillments, and not all wish fulfillments are sexual; many desires and forces drive us, from hunger to fear to love and friendship. This is a good example of a wish fulfillment dream.

A few years ago, I supervised a young trainee whom I greatly enjoyed. He was bright, motivated, and a pleasure to work with. Then he accepted a position at a university in the Midwest. Though happy for his success, I was sad to lose him here as a colleague. The night before he was scheduled to move, I dreamt that I was helping him load the moving van. As we filled the van with his furniture and belongings, each load seemed to get heavier and heavier. Finally, we packed up the last of his things and he hopped in the front seat to drive away. As he turned the key in the ignition, the truck would not start. Without a functioning moving van, he had to stay. Then I woke up.

Going through the same steps as before, we first assess the structure of the dream to determine whether or not it has a beginning, a middle, and an end. There is indeed a clear story within the dream: We first load up the truck, then the truck won't start, and finally, he does not move away. There are also some clear emotions in the dream. As the boxes get heavier and heavier to lift, I feel the growing sense of dread and sadness that he is going to move away. The elements in the dream about moving are clear day residue.

Finally, we look at the metaphors in the dream to interpret what it might mean. Given the context and the events leading up to the dream, one interpretation is that the moving truck is a metaphor for my true feelings about my friend moving away. As the time got closer for him to leave, I became sadder, just as the boxes became heavier. The failure of the truck's engine then represents my desire for him to stay. According to this metaphor, this is ultimately a dream about relationships, aging, separation, and the loss of a mentee.

Now, let's turn to examples from my students. Remember, when we analyze these dreams, we will find that each one fits into one of these grand themes:

- Birth
- Growing up
- Relationships
- Achievement
- Love
- Sickness
- Separation
- Loss
- Death.

Student 13—The horse

> There was a horse next to my house/office (not sure). All of a sudden the horse got released. Some of the people were enjoying this happening, but I was frightened. My former employee (the best sales guy I had in my previous business) appeared.

First, let's determine whether or not this dream has psychological significance. Is there a clear story? The events in the dream are not logically or temporally linked—it has no clear beginning, middle, or concluding action. A horse is released, but then the former employee appears, seemingly out of nowhere and without reason. There is emotionality present—the onlookers are happy, while the dreamer is frightened.

We cannot be sure whether or not it contains day residue. There does not seem to be an overarching metaphor, and the dream is difficult to place into one of the grand themes. This dream is likely not a reflection of unconscious processes and can be discarded as random neuronal discharges.

The length of the dream also indicates it is not meaningful. Notice how brief the recollection is compared to some of the dreams below. Typically, significant dreams are recalled and recorded in much greater detail than this one, and they produce a longer word count.

Student 14—History exam

> History phobia. The History exam is coming and there are only two weeks left. There are a lot of notes I haven't memorized yet and it makes me so nervous and desperate. I take all my history notes, from European History to Asian History, to school and revise. But I just can't memorize anything. Then, my teacher announces that there will be a History test and I feel like I'm going to die.

First, is the dream meaningful or not? There is a clear progression of events with a beginning, middle, and an end. A history exam is coming up, the student tries to study but can't remember anything, and her anxiety culminates when the teacher announces the test. This is a story. There is also a strong sense of anxiety, fear, and frustration. As outsiders we do not know if any day residue is present, but the clear story and strong emotionality are indicative of a psychologically meaningful dream.

Next, we look for the metaphor and see if we can place it within the grand themes. The history test is acting as a metaphor for achievement and success. The stress induced by not feeling prepared for the test and the fear of failing likely reflect some kind of stress this student is experiencing in waking life, perhaps anxiety over work commitments or a fear that she will not live up to expectations. The grand theme is achievement.

Student 15—High school reunion

> I was at a high school reunion, a special celebration for important people and ex-students. I felt inappropriately dressed (wearing jeans). I also tried to

> regain the feeling of being among friends. Some family members attended. I was very elegant and I didn't know many of the people. Some photos were taken and I felt disappointed when I didn't show up in any of the photos, despite seeing several of my friends. Later I went back to the apartment where I was staying. A cousin of mine had invited us over for dinner. I wasn't feeling very festive so I turned the invitation down, but upon seeing his disappointment I changed my mind. I also showed older photos of my high school to my sister and tried to explain where everything was today (the administrative building, the secretary's office, etc.). I remember seeing lots of natural settings in those photos (cows, mountains, hills, etc.). I liked the sight of those photos.

The story in this dream is straightforward. First she goes to the high school reunion. While there, she has various anxiety provoking experiences, and then she leaves and goes to her cousin's house for dinner. There is a clear sense of disappointment and stress caused by not fitting in, leading us to conclude that the dream does have meaningful unconscious roots.

The high school reunion is a metaphor for relationships and belonging, placing the dream in the affiliation category. High school is, stereotypically, a socially anxious time, and high school reunions are infamous for stirring up these anxious feelings and for creating a need to impress former classmates. There are a few different examples of the dreamer feeling like she does not fit in with the group, from wearing the wrong outfit to not showing up in the photographs. She wants to be a part of the group, but continues to feel like an outsider.

This same sentiment is expressed in a different way when, to please her cousin, she agrees to go to a dinner that she does not want to attend. Here our analysis becomes more nuanced, once we remember that she is the orchestrator of the dream. Her unconscious mind created this scenario and was in control of the other characters in the dream, their actions, and their feelings. If she unconsciously chose for her cousin to be disappointed when she initially turned down the dinner invitation, this could again reflect her desire to be wanted by others.

The only happiness expressed in the dream is when she looks at photographs of nature—photographs that contain no people to worry about fitting in with. The underlying meaning here reveals some discontent with her interpersonal relationships, a desire to fit in, and perhaps some social insecurity.

Student 16—Ghosts

> I am in my house/apartment with my parents, on a normal day. We are speaking or passing time together in the same room. Everything is fine. At some point I have to go to another room, which has only one door in common with the previous one. While I enter the room I see one of my parents in there, and this makes me feel anxious. It is not possible that my father/mother is in two places at the same time. This should be a ghost. I am afraid, even though the "new mother/father" does not look dangerous. I start screaming, calling the previous parent to see if he/she is still in the other room, trying to understand what is happening. Sometimes the sound does not come out, sometimes they answer from the previous room. But the one in the new room starts speaking normally as my parent would do, saying that he/she is real. But I know that he/she is not. I don't have to trust him/her. The anxiety and the fear increase. At this point I start to take control of the dream. I think that this can't happen in the reality and think that I am dreaming. So I try to convince myself to wake me up, just repeating to myself "Wake up, wake up!" till I do it.

With both a chronological story and clear emotionality, this dream is another example that contains underlying psychological meaning. The scene is set up with the narrator in a room with her parents. She then finds a duplicate of her parents in a second room, which creates confusion, anxiety, and fear. The story concludes when she realizes that the situation cannot be real, and she tries to wake up. There is a sense of growing unease and panic throughout the dream.

This dream is a metaphor for the dreamer's conflicted feelings about her parents, and the grand themes here are growing up and separation. On one hand, she is disturbed and frightened by the idea that her parents have turned into ghosts and cannot be trusted. Her fear heightens when she tries unsuccessfully to turn to them for reassurance and comfort. On the other hand, she has orchestrated a dream in which she has turned her parents into untrustworthy ghosts, revealing some desire to gain space from them. On this level, she does not want to rely on them for comfort. Her resolution for the situation is then to take control by forcing herself to wake up. While growing up and separating from her parents may be a scary idea, she simultaneously longs for independence and to be in control of her life.

Student 17—Great-grandfather

I saw a picture in a frame on a shelf and was totally upset about it. John, the boy who has a job on my dad's farm, was sitting on the lap of my great-grandfather who died ten years ago. The way he held him on his lap was the way he always used to hold me. It made me really mad and I couldn't understand it, because they have no relationship to each other and never met. I cried.

The story here is simple but clear—she sees a picture of John sitting on her great-grandfather's lap, which reminded her of the way her great-grandfather used to hold her, and she became upset. There are unquestionable emotions present. She describes being angry and confused by the photograph. This student explained that in waking life, her great-grandfather was "strong, smart, and very lovely" and an important part of the family. She also described how John works at her family farm daily helping her father, but that he acts more like a member of the family than an employee. A clear day residue is therefore present in the dream.

The dream is a metaphor for her rivalry with John. Her great-grandfather, the cornerstone of her family, holding John the way he used to hold her, indicates her concern over being replaced. Her feelings make sense, given that she reported that John is at her family's farm every day, spends a lot of time with her father, and acts more like family than an employee. Her emotional reaction to this scenario is also telling of her feelings about John. She does not want to be replaced by him and is perhaps upset by his closeness to her family. The overall theme is one of affiliation.

The final layer here is that she was the orchestrator of her dream: She chose to see a picture of John with her great-grandfather. She chose not to place herself on her great-grandfather's lap. She may have some conflicting emotions about her place in the family. Perhaps she does not want to be replaced by John, but, on another level, she also craves her own independence, away from her family.

Student 18—Waiting for the flight

This dream is a flash back to a situation which happened about 1965. In its opening I am looking out at skyline approach to Minneapolis airport awaiting

> arrival of a friend, Jane, who is relocating from her parents' home to take up employment there as flight attendant. My dream begins with my overview of skyline of Minneapolis airport. I remember awaiting there (in my car) for Jane's flight wondering where, if anywhere, this relationship might go. Her flight was somewhat late, so I languish on impatiently. Something about the impending anticipation has lingered on memorably for me. As it happens Jane's flight arrives anti-climatically late ... so we go on routinely.

This dream is both a story and emotionally charged. The scene is set with background information about Jane and the dreamer waiting for her flight. He wonders if the relationship will turn romantic and becomes impatient when her flight is delayed. The dream concludes with the arrival of her flight and with the two continuing as friends. There are feelings of impatience, anticipation, hopefulness, and ultimately disappointment.

At face value, this is a dream about the memory of dashed hopes. Travel is acting as a metaphor for love. The dreamer had anxiously anticipated the arrival of Jane's flight, wondering if the relationship might turn romantic, but the flight was late and an anticlimactic end left them as just friends. The dream is a rehearsal of this real life experience.

However, an unconscious layer is embedded beneath this surface level interpretation. His unconscious is in control of the dream; he wrote the script. He could have changed the scenario in any way he liked in order to fulfill his wishes. He could have had Jane's flight arrive on time, he could have lived out the fantasy of romance, he could even have married Jane if that is what he had hoped for. Instead, his unconscious chose to have the relationship remain platonic. He chose disappointment. Some part of him did not want the relationship to progress. The grand theme is love, and perhaps not wanting the complications of love.

Student 19—The zip line

> A man I used to have a crush on who used to live in the city said to me to try zip lining in San Francisco—that they have the highest view from the trees (or something cryptic to this effect). I got up to this contraption that was a zip line with just a handle bar without any seats, straps, or security. I knew it was a long way to the other side—I could see the end. I thought, "How can I hold myself up? I don't know if I'm strong enough." Still, I grabbed

> the bar on both ends. I looked down, and indeed, it seemed very high. The more I touched the bars and looked down, the higher I seemed. At one point the ground looked so far away, it was as if I were looking down from an airplane. Then, my vision focused again to a lower level. I saw several tall trees below me, and directly underneath the zip line path were train tracks. Somehow I knew I would be okay. I don't remember the release, but I do remember being in the air. There were some other people on their own zip lines going in several different directions, too. It was a quick "flight" but I made it to the other side. I think I was met by that man, where he said, "See? I knew it could be done." It wasn't an overly triumphant feeling, but I realized when I woke up that I was strong enough to cross to the other side of San Francisco.

This a structured story with a beginning, middle, and end. There is a progression of emotions, from nervousness and fear in the beginning, to a calm confidence by the end. The zip line is acting as a metaphor for conquering an obstacle. At first, it seems insurmountable—the zip line feels too high and too long—and she doubts her capability. Then, she finds confidence in herself and takes the plunge, successfully making it to the other side of the city.

Given the use of a zip line over San Francisco and the presence of a former crush, this dream may be a metaphor for the difficulties that accompany living in a big city or for romantic relationships. It could be a metaphor for many different situations that involve facing challenges, and the correct interpretation will depend on the dreamer's waking life circumstances. Overall, this is a dream about succeeding, daring to take risks, and needing some encouragement to do so.

Our dreams can contain a wealth of insight into who we are and what we want. With an understanding of which dreams merit attention and how to approach the analysis, we can decode our dream lives and unearth our deep desires, fears, thoughts, and emotions. The unconscious speaks to us every night; all we have to do is learn the language of dreams, and listen. In doing so, as is so often seen in clinical practice, we gain an understanding of our behaviors, desires, and decisions, and gain the power to make changes towards a healthier, happier life.

Memes, slips, art analysis, expressive writing, and dream analysis all have unique benefits and will appeal differently to each of us: Some may find that they learn the most about themselves through their dreams, while others may find expressive writing to be a more helpful tool.

Whatever path we choose, learning what sleeping dogs are lurking in our unconscious and how they affect our lives allows us to make important changes. Sometimes, sleeping dogs do just sleep. But more often, they nip at our heels and push us in directions that we don't necessarily want to go. These five channels of access to the unconscious mind give us back the power to choose our own directions—and to have some fun while we are doing it.

EPILOGUE

Rainer Maria Rilke (1997) once said, "I live my life in widening circles that reach out across the world." This should be the final mantra, as we finish this journey into our unconscious mind. We have reached the end point of a long and increasingly intensifying exploration of your deeper self. Along the way, I have given you several tools to help you appreciate art, music, and writing from a new perspective. These tools can also show you aspects of yourself that you may not have recognized. Some discoveries may be surprising, and some may be more like old friends that you have not visited in a while. Some may be positive, and others negative and not necessarily desirable.

The exercises I have discussed allow you to examine who you are and who you want to be. At the very least, you will find that your view of who you are will have expanded considerably and that new opportunities for growth are now within your grasp.

How do my students benefit from this intensive self-examination? While I have no controlled follow-up studies, I do have impressions gathered over the past decade of teaching this course. Almost inevitably, a bonding forms within the class. Relationships emerge and persist beyond the duration of the course, and the atmosphere during class becomes protective and supportive, fostering a sense of safety for self-exploration. Some students return for more instruction along the same lines, and some even return with a friend or partner to retake the class.

Many students begin to appreciate talents that they had previously under-appreciated, leading to an examination of career trajectories and choices. Often they rediscover their artistic creativity, which at the beginning of class had been faltering under the impact of the debris of life. Others report a renewed appreciation of art, music, and writing.

Some students find that issues that arose earlier in their lives are still adversely affecting them, and they return to psychiatric or psychological treatment to rework those issues. Most of these students find the class helpful in defining what help they need to return to symptom-free functioning and continued personal growth.

Ultimately, I hope that you receive these same benefits. In the past decade, a humanistic perspective has become more prominent in the practice of medicine and psychiatry. Instead of the traditional view of the super-expert doctor, a humanistic perspective puts the individual in charge of himself. The motivation behind offering this class and writing this book is in line with these humanistic efforts. Our goal is to offer you the opportunity to examine your own life, make you the expert of your own life, and put you in control of your choices, reactions, and emotions.

APPENDIX

This appendix contains the screens and scoring information discussed in Chapter Three. You may copy and use them for your own personal use. For more extensive use in a clinic or for research, please contact Dr. Steiner for permission via his website: www.hanssteiner.com.

In case you decide to have us help you interpret or maybe even publish your results, we have also included a consent form. This form only needs to be signed and returned to us if you would like help with your results. For more information, please contact Becky via her website: www.rebeccahall.net. If you work at another academic institution, you may have your own version of this consent form.

General Health Questionnaire 30 (GHQ30)

Please go to the following website to purchase a copy of the GHQ30: https://shop.acer.edu.au/ghq-30-item-questionnaire-ghq-30.

To score your completed GHQ, the two most symptomatic answers for each question score a "1" (the two right hand columns), and the two least symptomatic answers score a "0" (the two left hand columns). Add the scores for each question together for your total score. In this simple scoring pattern, any answer on the left side of the page gets a "0," and any on the right side of the page gets a "1." There are more detailed and complicated methods of scoring this scale that can be obtained by consulting the articles listed in the further reading section on Dr. Steiner's website (details given at the start of the References).

Facts About You questionnaire (FAY)

1. Are you: _______ MALE _______ FEMALE

2. What is your ethnic background?

   _______ AFRICAN AMERICAN _______ HISPANIC _______ ASIAN

   _______ WHITE _______ NATIVE AMERICAN _______ OTHER

3. Your AGE: _____ 4. Does your family usually speak English at home? ___ YES ___ NO

5. Your date of birth is: ___ / ___ / ___

6. I have finished: (check one)

   ___ (1) ELEMENTARY SCHOOL

   ___ (2) MIDDLE/JR. HIGH SCHOOL

   ___ (3) HIGH SCHOOL

   ___ (4) JUNIOR COLLEGE

   ___ (5) COLLEGE

   ___ (6) GRADUATE DEGREE (MA, PhD, MD)

7. My Partner has finished: (check one)

   ___ (1) ELEMENTARY SCHOOL

   ___ (2) MIDDLE/JR. HIGH SCHOOL

   ___ (3) HIGH SCHOOL

   ___ (4) JUNIOR COLLEGE

   ___ (5) COLLEGE

   ___ (6) GRADUATE DEGREE (MA, PhD, MD)

8. I work as a: (fill in the blank) ______________________________

9. My partner works as a: (fill in the blank) ______________________________

10. Do you have any serious or long term health problems? (circle one) YES NO

11. What are they? ______________________________

12. How many times have you had to stay in the hospital (circle one)

    NEVER 1 TIME 2–6 TIMES 7 or MORE TIMES

13. What for? ______________________________

14. How happy are you with each of the following areas of your life? (circle one)

SCHOOL/WORK	very UNhappy	1	2	3	4	5	6	7	8	9	very happy
FRIENDS	very UNhappy	1	2	3	4	5	6	7	8	9	very happy
FAMILY	very UNhappy	1	2	3	4	5	6	7	8	9	very happy
FREE TIME	very UNhappy	1	2	3	4	5	6	7	8	9	very happy

16. Have you ever gone to a counselor/psychologist/psychiatrist? (circle one) YES NO

17. Are you now going to a counselor/psychologist/psychiatrist? (circle one) YES NO

18. If yes, for how long did you see/are you seeing this person? (circle one)

    3 months or less 4–12 months 13 months or more

19. In general, how happy are you with yourself?

    very UNhappy 1 2 3 4 5 6 7 8 9 very happy

Facts About You population means

	Population mean	*Standard deviation*	*1 Standard deviation range*	*½ Standard deviation*	*½ Standard deviation range*
Happiness with Family	7.1	2.0	5.1–9.0	1.0	6.1–8.1
Happiness with Friends	7.4	1.8	5.6–9.0	0.9	6.5–8.3
Happiness with Work	6.2	2.1	4.1–8.3	1.1	5.1–7.3
Happiness with Recreation	7.0	2.0	5.0–9.0	1.0	6.0–8.0
Overall Happiness	7.0	1.8	5.2–8.8	0.9	6.1–7.9

Weinberger Adjustment Inventory questionnaire (WAI-84)

Name__________ Date__________

WAI-84

The purpose of these questions is to understand what you are *usually* like or what you have *usually* felt, not just during the past few weeks but over the *past year* or more.

Please read each sentence carefully and circle the number that best describes you. For each sentence in Part I, decide whether it is: (1) *false or mostly false,* (2) *somewhat false,* (I.e., more false than true); (4) *somewhat true,* (I.e., more true than false); or (5) *true or mostly true* for you. If you can't really say that it's more true or more false, circle (3) for *not sure.*

Example: If the question were: "I spend a lot of time reading," and you read some but not that much, you would circle (2) *somewhat false.*

Part I	*FALSE*	*Somewhat FALSE*	*Not sure*	*Somewhat TRUE*	*TRUE*
1. I enjoy most of the things I do during the week.	1	2	3	4	5
2. There have been times when I said I would do one thing but did something else.	1	2	3	4	5
3. I often feel that nobody really cares about me the way I want them to.	1	2	3	4	5
4. Doing things to help other people is more important to me than almost anything else.	1	2	3	4	5
5. I spend a lot of time thinking about things that might go wrong.	1	2	3	4	5
6. There are times when I'm not very proud of how well I've done something.	1	2	3	4	5
7. No matter what I'm doing, I usually have a good time.	1	2	3	4	5

Part I	*FALSE*	*Somewhat FALSE*	*Not sure*	*Somewhat TRUE*	*TRUE*
8. I'm the kind of person who will try anything once, even if it's no that safe.	1	2	3	4	5
9. I'm not very sure of myself.	1	2	3	4	5
10. Some things have happened this year that I felt unhappy about at the time	1	2	3	4	5
11. Once in a while. I don't do something that someone asked me to do.	1	2	3	4	5
12. I can remember a time when I was so angry at someone that I felt like hurting them.	1	2	3	4	5
13. I am answering these questions truthfully.	1	2	3	4	5
14. In recent years, there have been a lot of times when I've felt unhappy and down about things.	1	2	3	4	5
15. I usually think of myself as a happy person.	1	2	3	4	5
16. I have done some things that weren't right and felt sorry about it later.	1	2	3	4	5
17. I usually don't let things upset me too much.	1	2	3	4	5
18. I can think of times when I did not feel very good about myself.	1	2	3	4	5
19. I should try harder to control myself when I'm having fun.	1	2	3	4	5
20. I do things that are against the law more often than most people.	1	2	3	4	5
21. I really don't like myself very much.	1	2	3	4	5
22. I usually have a great time when I do things with other people.	1	2	3	4	5
23. When I try something for the first time, I am always sure I'll be good at it.	1	2	3	4	5

Part I	*FALSE*	*Somewhat FALSE*	*Not sure*	*Somewhat TRUE*	*TRUE*
24. I never feel sad about things that happen to me.	1	2	3	4	5
25. I never act like I know more about something than I really do.	1	2	3	4	5
26. I often go out of my way to do things for other people.	1	2	3	4	5
27. I sometimes feel so bad about myself that I wish I were somebody else.	1	2	3	4	5
28. I'm the kind of person who smiles and laughs a lot.	1	2	3	4	5
29. Once in a while, I say bad things about people that I would not say in front of them.	1	2	3	4	5
30. Once in a while, I break a promise I've made.	1	2	3	4	5
31. Once in a while, I get upset about something that I later see was not that important.	1	2	3	4	5
32. Everyone makes mistakes at least once in a while.	1	2	3	4	5
33. Most of the time, I really don't worry about things very much.	1	2	3	4	5
34. I'm the kind of person who has a lot of fun.	1	2	3	4	5
35. I often feel like not trying anymore because I can't seem to make things better.	1	2	3	4	5
36. People who get me angry better watch out.	1	2	3	4	5
37. There have been times when I did not finish something because I spent too much time goofing off.	1	2	3	4	5
38. I worry too much about things that aren't' important.	1	2	3	4	5
39. There have been times when I didn't let people know about something I did wrong.	1	2	3	4	5

Part I	*FALSE*	*Somewhat FALSE*	*Not sure*	*Somewhat TRUE*	*TRUE*
40. I am never unkind to people I don't like.	1	2	3	4	5
41. I sometimes give up doing something because I don't think I am very good at it.	1	2	3	4	5
42. I often feel sad or unhappy.	1	2	3	4	5
43. Once in a while, I say things that aren't completely true.	1	2	3	4	5
44. I usually feel I'm the kind of person I want to be.	1	2	3	4	5
45. I have never met anyone younger than I am.	1	2	3	4	5

The questions in Part II relate to how *often* you think, feel or act a certain way. Again, we want to know What is usual for you even if it hasn't happened in the past couple of days or weeks. After you read each sentence carefully, please *circle* how often it is true: (1) *almost never or never*, (2) *not often*, (3) *sometimes* or an average amount, (4) *often*, or (5) *almost always*.

Part II	*Never*	*Not often*	*Some-times*	*Often*	*Almost always*
46. I feel I can do things as well as other people.	1	2	3	4	5
47. I think about other people's feelings before I do something they might not like.	1	2	3	4	5
48. I do things without giving them enough thought.	1	2	3	4	5
49. When I have the chance, I take things I want that don't really belong to me.	1	2	3	4	5
50. If someone tries to hurt me, I make sure I get even with them.	1	2	3	4	5
51. I enjoy doing things for other people, even when I don't receive anything in return.	1	2	3	4	5
52. I feel afraid if I think someone might hurt me.	1	2	3	4	5
53. I get into such a bad mood that I feel like just sitting around and doing nothing.	1	2	3	4	5
54. I become "wild and crazy" and do things other people might not like.	1	2	3	4	5
55. I do things that are really not fair to people I don't care about.	1	2	3	4	5
56. I will cheat on something if I know no one will find out.	1	2	3	4	5
57. When I'm doing something for fun (for example, partying, acting silly), I tend to get carried away and go too far.	1	2	3	4	5

Part II	*Never*	*Not often*	*Some-times*	*Often*	*Almost always*
58. I feel very happy.	1	2	3	4	5
59. I make sure that doing what I want will not cause problems for other people.	1	2	3	4	5
60. I break laws and rules I don't agree with.	1	2	3	4	5
61. I feel at least a little upset when people point out things I have done wrong.	1	2	3	4	5
62. I feel that I am a special or important person.	1	2	3	4	5
63. I like to do new and different things that many people would consider weird or not really safe.	1	2	3	4	5
64. I get nervous when I know I need to do my best (on a job, team, etc.)	1	2	3	4	5
65. Before I do something, I think about how it will affect the people around me.	1	2	3	4	5
66. If someone does something I really don't like, I yell at them about it.	1	2	3	4	5
67. People can depend on me to do what I know I should.	1	2	3	4	5
68. I lose my temper and "let people have it" when I'm angry.	1	2	3	4	5
69. I feel so down and unhappy that nothing makes me feel much better.	1	2	3	4	5
70. In recent years. I have felt more nervous or worried about things than I have needed to.	1	2	3	4	5
71. I do things that I know really aren't right.	1	2	3	4	5

Part II	*Never*	*Not often*	*Some-times*	*Often*	*Almost always*
72. I say the first thing that comes into my mind without thinking enough about it.	1	2	3	4	5
73. I pick on people I don't like.	1	2	3	4	5
74. I feel afraid something terrible might happen to me or someone I care about.	1	2	3	4	5
75. I feel a little down when I don't do as well as I thought I would.	1	2	3	4	5
76. If people I like do things without asking me to join them, I feel, a little left out.	1	2	3	4	5
77. I try very hard not to hurt other people's feelings.	1	2	3	4	5
78. I feel nervous or afraid that things won't work out the way I would like them to.	1	2	3	4	5
79. I stop and think things through before I act.	1	2	3	4	5
80. I say something mean to someone who has upset me.	1	2	3	4	5
81. I make sure I stay out of trouble.	1	2	3	4	5
82. I feel lonely.	1	2	3	4	5
83. I feel that I am really good at things I try to do.	1	2	3	4	5
84. When someone tries to start a fight with me, I fight back.	1	2	3	4	5

Did you answer all of the questions?
Thank you!

Weinberger Adjustment Inventory (WAI-84) scoring instructions

Using the formulas below, you can create a score sheet in Excel. Then, calculate your score for each variable and compare your score to your age-matched mean. A difference of 0.5 between your score and the age-matched mean, either above or below, is considered significant. In each formula, "Qx" represents your score for "question x." For example, if you rated your answer to question number five as "3," you would input "3" in place of "Q5" into the formulas below.

Population means for the WAI variables

	Your score	*Ages 11–12*	*Ages 13–16*	*Ages 17–30*	*Ages 31–60*
Distress		2.7	2.6	2.6	2.2
Anxiety		2.9	2.9	2.8	2.6
Anger		2.5	2.4	2.4	1.9
Depression		2.7	2.6	2.6	2.2
Positive Emotions		3.8	3.9	3.9	4.1
Happiness		4.0	3.9	3.9	3.9
Self-Esteem		3.6	3.8	3.8	4.2
Restraint		3.7	3.7	3.6	4.1
Impulse Control		3.5	3.5	3.4	4.0
Consideration of Others		3.5	3.7	3.6	3.9
Responsibility		4.2	4.0	3.9	4.5
Repressive Defensiveness		2.4	2.3	2.4	3.0
Denial of Distress		2.5	2.3	2.4	2.7

1. Validity Score = [Q13 + Q32 + (6-Q45)]/3
   a. This score must be 3.7 or more in all age groups in order for your results to be valid. If your Validity Score is below 3.7, please retake the questionnaire.
2. Anxiety = [Q5 + (6-Q17) + (6-Q33) + Q38 + Q64 + Q70 + Q74 + Q78]/8
3. Anger = (Q36 + Q50 + Q66 + Q68 + Q73 + Q80 + Q84)/7
4. Depression = (Q3 + Q14 + Q35 + Q42 + Q53 + Q69 + Q82)/7

5. Happiness = (Q1 + Q7 + Q15 + Q22 + Q28 + Q34 + Q58)/7
6. Self-Esteem = [(6-Q9) + (6-Q21) + (6-Q27) + Q44 + Q46 + Q62 + Q83]/7
7. Impulse Control = [(6-Q8) + (6-Q19) + (6-Q48) + (6-Q54) + (6-Q57) + (6-Q63) + (6-Q72) + Q79]/8
8. Consideration of Others = (Q4 + Q26 + Q47 + Q51 + Q59 + Q65 + Q77)/7
9. Responsibility = [(6-Q20) + (6-Q49) + (6-Q55) + (6-Q56) + (6-Q60) + Q67 + (6-Q71) + Q81]/8
10. Repressive Defensiveness = [(6-Q2) + (6-Q11) – (6-Q12) + (6-Q16) + Q25 + (6-Q29) + (6-Q30) + (6-Q37) + (6-Q39) + Q40 + (6-Q43)]/11
11. Denial of Distress = [(6-Q6) + (6-Q10) + (6-Q18) + Q23 + Q24 + (6-Q31) + (6-Q41) + (6-Q52) + (6-Q61) + (6-Q75) + (6-Q76)]/11

Composite Scores

1. Distress = (Anxiety score + Anger score + Depression score)/3
2. Positive Emotions = (Happiness score + Self-Esteem score)/2
3. Restraint = (Impulse Control score + Consideration of Others score + Responsibility score)/3

Response Evaluation Measure questionnaire (REM-71)

REM-71

Please read each of the statements on this questionnaire and, as you read each one, think about how true it is of you during the past few months. You can mark how much you think the statement is true of you on the separate response sheet or on the questionnaire.

FOR EXAMPLE

	STRONGLY DISAGREE		NOT SURE		STRONGLY AGREE
I have dark brown hair	1	3	5	7	9

If your hair is dark brown, you would write "9" on the answer sheet. If it is some shade or mixture of brown, you would write a lower number. If it has no brown, you would write "1".

ANOTHER EXAMPLE

	STRONGLY DISAGREE		NOT SURE		STRONGLY AGREE
I have not met anyone younger than I am.	1	3	5	7	9

You would probably write a "1" on the response sheet!

If you have any questions, just ask the person who is working with you.

Thank you for your cooperation.

Division of Child Psychiatry
401 Quarry Road
Stanford, CA 94305-5719

REF: Steiner, H., & Feldman, S. S. (1995). Two approaches to the measure of adaptive style: Comparison of normal, psychosomatically ill, and delinquent adolescents. *Journal of the American Academy of Child and Adolescent Psychiatry, 34*(2): 180–190.

Feldman, S. S., Araujo, K., & Steiner, H. (1996). Defense mechanisms in adolescents as a function of age, sex, and mental health status. *Journal of the American Academy of Child and Adolescent Psychiatry, 35*: 1344–1354.

Steiner, H., Araujo, K., & Koopman, C. (2001). The response evaluation measure: A new instrument for the assessment of defenses *American Journal of Psychiatry, 158*(3): 467–473.

REM-71

STRONGLY DISAGREE		NOT SURE		STRONGLY AGREE
1	3	5	7	9

1. Discussing disagreements with my family usually helps.
2. I usually use my head and do not "go with my gut."
3. When I get stressed I get ill really easily.
4. I go out of my way to help people.
5. I don't want to brag, but usually I'm the one who knows how to get things done.
6. When I am upset I remind myself that everything is really okay.
7. I laugh at myself pretty easily.
8. If someone is unfair to me I probably won't do what I told them I'd do.
9. I often get very upset with people even though they haven't really bothered me.
10. When things upset me I'd rather be by myself.
11. When I don't like someone I try hard not to get angry at them.
12. I know this great person whose advice I can usually trust.
13. I like to write stories or poems when I've just been through a really rough situation.
14. I have lost my voice or sight or hearing for a long time and the doctors didn't know why.
15. I often get the feeling that whatever is going on is not really happening to me.
16. Some of the worst things which happen to me make funny stories later.
17. Often I act really nice when actually I'm pretty upset.
18. A lot of people I know don't appreciate how gifted and great I am.
19. I often agree to do a job, but then I somehow just don't get around to it.
20. People tell me that I don't show my true feelings.

STRONGLY DISAGREE		NOT SURE		STRONGLY AGREE
1	3	5	7	9

21. I have had trouble walking or using my hands and doctors couldn't find anything wrong with me.
22. Helping others is very important to me.
23. When I do certain things in exactly the right way it keeps bad things from happening.
24. I won't let people in authority know I'm angry at them, but everyone else better watch out!
25. I get a headache when I have to do something I don't like to do.
26. I know a wonderful person who understands me perfectly and will not hurt me.
27. Often, things which worry or frighten other people don't really bother me at all.
28. I usually try to help people when they have problems.
29. Sometimes I have lost all the feeling in one part of my body and nobody could explain why.
30. When things go wrong I can still see the funny side.
31. Sometimes people think I am upset when I know I'm not.
32. Everyone is against me.
33. I often do things without thinking first.
34. I handle problems by staying calm.
35. There are some shows, where I like to imagine that I am in the story.
36. Some people act really nice, but later they prove what jerks they are.
37. When I should have strong feelings, I don't feel anything.
38. I am often treated unfairly.
39. I don't get upset during arguments because I just look at things logically.
40. When things get really tense, I tell myself that it's no big deal.

STRONGLY DISAGREE		NOT SURE		STRONGLY AGREE
1	3	5	7	9

41. I repeat special thoughts or words over and over to myself when I am uptight or frightened.
42. People should stay the same, instead of being nice one day and completely the opposite the next.
43. I think it's really important to help people who have problems.
44. When things bother me I find something creative to do.
45. I have usually told the absolute truth.
46. I know someone who has such wonderful wisdom and ability that they can handle any problem perfectly.
47. I use reason and logic, not feelings, to understand people.
48. If I don't like someone, I'll be extra nice to them.
49. When I'm in stressful situations I often space out.
50. When I'm upset or angry I do things without thinking.
51. I usually see a funny side to the problems I have.
52. When I'm in an argument, I try to think clearly and do not get upset.
53. I like to listen to music that fits my mood.
54. When I'm upset, I try to be alone and not talk to anyone.
55. I often get so carried away that my friends have to help me calm down.
56. I often do special things to bring me good luck.
57. When I need to, I can put my problems on hold until later when I can think about them.
58. I feel like somebody is out to get me.
59. Role-playing games are a good way to feel like I am really someone else.
60. When someone bothers me I talk to them and explain how I feel.

STRONGLY DISAGREE		NOT SURE		STRONGLY AGREE
1	3	5	7	9

61. When someone I like lets me down, I do not trust them again.
62. If I had a chance, I could do a better job than most people around me.
63. When I can't get out of doing something, I usually just do it slowly.
64. I can keep my problems out of my mind until I have time to deal with them.
65. When someone makes me angry, I might wreck something of theirs.
66. I have found myself in places and had no idea how I got there.
67. I like to imagine that my life is very different.
68. If someone bothers me, I usually just talk to them about it and things work out.
69. I usually find a way to be alone when I'm unhappy.
70. When I get stressed I get a stomachache.
71. I enjoy most of what I do every day.

Did you respond to each statement? Thank You!

Response Evaluation Measure (REM-71) scoring instructions

Using the formulas below, you can create an Excel score sheet. Then, calculate your score for each variable and compare your score to your age-matched mean. A difference of 0.5 between your score and the age-matched mean, above or below, is considered significant. In each formula, "Qx" represents your score for "question x." For example, if you rated your answer to question number five as a "3," you would input a 3 in place of "Q5" into the formulas below.

Population means for the REM-71 variables

	Your score	*Adolescent mean*	*20–39 mean*	*40+ mean*
Factor 1 Interpersonal		4.1	2.8	2.5
Acting Out		4.8	3.8	3.3
Displacement		3.9	1.7	1.7
Passive Aggression		4.9	3.1	2.9
Projection		3.0	1.7	1.5
Splitting		5.6	3.7	3.7
Withdrawal		5.9	5.4	5.3
Factor 1 Intrapsychic		3.9	3.7	3.4
Conversion		1.6	1.2	1.4
Dissociation		3.9	2.8	2.4
Fantasy		4.6	3.9	3.3
Omnipotence		5.7	5.2	4.8
Repression		4.9	4.5	4.2
Somatization		3.8	3.7	3.5
Sublimation		5.5	4.7	4.3
Undoing		4.6	3.5	3.4
Factor 2 Interpersonal		5.3	5.3	5.4
Altruism		6.8	5.9	5.6
Humor		5.4	6.8	6.8
Idealization		5.7	3.8	4.6
Reaction Formation		4.5	4.7	4.5

	Your score	*Adolescent mean*	*20–39 mean*	*40+ mean*
Factor 2 Intrapsychic		4.5	5.4	5.4
Denial		5.1	5.8	5.4
Intellectualization		4.6	4.9	5.1
Suppression		4.8	5.4	5.6
Neutral				
Factor 1 Assimilation		4.5	3.5	3.2
Factor 2 Accommodation		5.3	5.4	5.5

1. Acting Out = (Q33 + Q50 + Q55)/3
2. Displacement = (Q9 + Q24 + Q65)/3
3. Passive Aggression = (Q8 + Q19 + Q63)/3
4. Projection = (Q32 + Q38 + Q58)/3
5. Splitting = (Q36 + Q42 + Q61)/3
6. Withdrawal = (Q10 + Q54 + Q69)/3
7. Conversion = (Q14 + Q21 + Q29)/3
8. Dissociation = (Q15 + Q49 + Q66)/3
9. Fantasy = (Q35 + Q59 + Q67)/3
10. Omnipotence = (Q5+ Q18 + Q62)/3
11. Repression = (Q20 + Q31 + Q37)/3
12. Somatization = (Q3 + Q25 + Q70)/3
13. Sublimation = (Q13 + Q44 + Q53)/3
14. Undoing = (Q23 + Q41 + Q56)/3
15. Altruism = (Q4 + Q22 + Q28 + Q43)/4
16. Humor = (Q7 + Q16 + Q30 + Q51)/4
17. Idealization = (Q12 + Q26 + Q46)/3
18. Reaction Formation = (Q11 + Q17 + Q48)/3
19. Denial = (Q6 + Q27 + Q40)/3
20. Intellectualization = (Q2 + Q39 + Q47 + Q52)/4

21. Suppression = (Q34 + Q57 + Q64)/3
22. Neutral = (Q1 + Q45 + Q60 + Q68 + Q71)/5

Composite Scores

1. Factor 1 Interpersonal = (Acting Out + Displacement + Passive Aggression + Projection + Splitting + Withdrawal)/6
2. Factor 1 Intrapsychic = (Conversion + Dissociation + Fantasy + Omnipotence + Repression + Somatization + Sublimation + Undoing)/8
3. Factor 2 Interpersonal = (Altruism + Humor + Idealization + Reaction Formation)/4
4. Factor 2 Intrapsychic = (Denial + Intellectualization + Suppression)/3

Total Factor 1 and Factor 2 Scores

1. Factor 1 Assimilation = (Factor 1 Interpersonal + Factor 1 Intrapsychic)/2
2. Factor 2 Accommodation = (Factor 2 Interpersonal + Factor 2 Intrapsychic)/2

CONSENT

Date: ______________________

AUTHORIZATION TO USE CASE MATERIAL FOR PROFESSIONAL PUBLICATION AND RESEARCH

THIS IS A CONSENT AND RELEASE—PLEASE READ CAREFULLY.

Thank you for allowing me (Hans Steiner, M.D.) to use case material from your mental health assessment and treatment in publications intended primarily for the audience described below (hereinafter referred to as the Work). This letter serves as our complete agreement.

You consent to the possible use of transcripts of your sessions or other case material in the Work.

In no event will your name or address be used. If you so direct below, I will take reasonable and customary steps to change or remove data that in your and my judgment may be likely to enable you to be identified, but you understand that despite these efforts some detail may appear in the Work that could be considered to identify you. The use of this material is limited to clinical research and publication intended primarily for professionals in mental health and behavioral science and interested lay audiences.

Of course, the requirements of editing and preservation of context are such that submitted materials may be edited, but I will attempt to ensure that there is no material change in the submission. In addition, I will be taking reasonable and customary steps to delete identifying details.

Neither I, nor the Publisher of the Work, nor anyone engaged to perform services with respect to the Work shall be liable to you for any matter arising out of the participation described in this consent.

There are no agreements between us other than this one. This agreement can be changed only by a signed document. You understand that my publisher and I will be relying upon this release in proceeding to publication, and you should therefore consider it carefully.

Your signature below indicates your agreement to the above terms. Please sign both copies and return one to me, keeping the other for your records. Thank you for your participation in this project.

______________________	______________________
(Signature)	(Street Address)
______________________	______________________
(Name – please print clearly)	(City, State, Zip)
______________________	______________________
(Name of Clinician: Hans Steiner, M.D.)	(Signature of Clinician, Hans Steiner, M.D.)

CHECK IF "YES"
( ) Detail deemed to be identifying to be changed or deleted: ______________

____
(Signature)

If under age 18, or otherwise deemed to be necessary or advisable:

______________________	______________________
(Name of Legal Guardian)	(Signature of Legal Guardian)

Date: ____________

CONSENT

Date: ____________________

AUTHORIZATION TO USE CASE MATERIAL FOR PROFESSIONAL PUBLICATION AND RESEARCH

THIS IS A CONSENT AND RELEASE—PLEASE READ CAREFULLY.

Thank you for allowing me (Hans Steiner, M.D.) to use case material from your mental health assessment and treatment in publications intended primarily for the audience described below (hereinafter referred to as the Work). This letter serves as our complete agreement.

You consent to the possible use of transcripts of your sessions or other case material in the Work.

In no event will your name or address be used. If you so direct below, I will take reasonable and customary steps to change or remove data that in your and my judgment may be likely to enable you to be identified, but you understand that despite these efforts some detail may appear in the Work that could be considered to identify you. The use of this material is limited to clinical research and publication intended primarily for professionals in mental health and behavioral science and interested lay audiences.

Of course, the requirements of editing and preservation of context are such that submitted materials may be edited, but I will attempt to ensure that there is no material change in the submission. In addition, I will be taking reasonable and customary steps to delete identifying details.

Neither I, nor the Publisher of the Work, nor anyone engaged to perform services with respect to the Work shall be liable to you for any matter arising out of the participation described in this consent.

There are no agreements between us other than this one. This agreement can be changed only by a signed document. You understand that my publisher and I will be relying upon this release in proceeding to publication, and you should therefore consider it carefully.

Your signature below indicates your agreement to the above terms. Please sign both copies and return one to me, keeping the other for your records. Thank you for your participation in this project.

____________________	____________________
(Signature)	(Street Address)
____________________	____________________
(Name – please print clearly)	(City, State, Zip)
____________________	____________________
(Name of Clinician: Hans Steiner, M.D.)	(Signature of Clinician, Hans Steiner, M.D.)

CHECK IF "YES"

( ) Detail deemed to be identifying to be changed or deleted: ____________________

____

(Signature)

If under age 18, or otherwise deemed to be necessary or advisable:

____________________	____________________
(Name of Legal Guardian)	(Signature of Legal Guardian)

Date: ____________________

REFERENCES

The reader is also invited to visit Dr. Steiner's website (http://www.hanssteiner.com/books-by-dr-steiner/) for additional suggested readings on the topics covered in *Your Secret Mind*. The list of readings is reached through a link embedded in the description of the book. This web version of suggested further readings is updated regularly, keeping the reader informed of the most recent developments.

Anderson, M. C., Ochsner, K. N., Kuhl, B., Cooper, J., Robertson, E., Gabrieli, S. W., Glover, G. H., & Gabrieli, J. D. (2004). Neural systems underlying the suppression of unwanted memories. *Science, 303*(5655): 232–235.

Artemisia (1997). [Motion picture.] C. Hahnheiser, C. Airoldi, D. Workmann, & L. Pescarolo (Producers), A. Merlet (Director). United States: Miramax.

Artemisia: Una Donna Appassionata (2012). [Motion picture.] Milan, Italy: 24 Ore Cultura.

Aserinsky, E., & Kleitman, N. (1953). Regularly occurring periods of eye motility, and concomitant phenomena, during sleep. *Science, 118*(3062): 273–274.

Bandura, A. (1997). *Self-Efficacy: The Exercise of Control*. New York: W. H. Freeman.

Bargh, J. (2007). *Social Psychology and the Unconscious: The Automaticity of Higher Mental Processes*. New York: Psychology Press.

Barrett, C. (1966). Conversations on Freud. In: C. Barrett (Ed.), *Wittgenstein: Lectures & Conversations* (pp. 41–52). Berkeley, CA: University of California Press.

Barzini, L. (1983). *The Europeans*. New York: Simon & Schuster.

Barzini, L. (1996). *The Italians*. New York: Touchstone.

Bower, G. H. (1981). Mood and memory. *American Psychologist, 36*(2): 129–148.

Bucci, W., & Maskit, B. (2006). A weighted dictionary for referential activity. In: J. G. Shanahan, Y. Qu, & J. Wiebe (Eds.), *Computing Attitude and Affect in Text* (pp. 49–60). Dordrecht, The Netherlands: Springer.

Buckner, R. L., Andrews-Hanna, J. R., & Schacter, D. L. (2008). The brain's default network: anatomy, function, and relevance to disease. *Annals of the New York Academy of Sciences, 1124*: 1–38.

Burton, R. A. (2016, September 5). A life of meaning (reason not required). *The New York Times*. Retrieved from http://www.nytimes.com/2016/09/05/opinion/a-life-of-meaning-reason-not-required.html?mwrsm=Email

Carroll, S. (2016). *The Big Picture: On the Origins of Life, Meaning, and the Universe Itself*. New York: Dutton.

Cavalli-Sforza, L. L., Feldman, M. W., Chen, K. H., & Dornbusch, S. M. (1982). Theory and observation in cultural transmission. *Science, 218*(4567): 19–27.

Coetzee, J. M., & Kurtz, A. (2015). *The Good Story: Exchanges on Truth, Fiction, and Psychotherapy*. New York: Viking.

Cohen, E. S. (2000). The trials of Artemisia Gentileschi: A rape as history. *The Sixteenth Century Journal, 31*(1): 47–75.

Colapinto, J. (2007, April 16). The interpreter. *The New Yorker*. Retrieved from http://www.newyorker.com/magazine/2007/04/16/the-interpreter-2

Crick, F., & Mitchison, G. (1983). The function of dream sleep. *Nature, 304*(5922): 111–114.

Crowley, J. (May 2015). An artist of the sleeping world. *Harper's Magazine*. Retrieved from http://harpers.org/archive/2015/05/an-artist-of-the-sleeping-world/

Dawkins, R. (1976). *The Selfish Gene*. New York: Oxford University Press.

De Mente, B. L. (2003). *Kata: The Key to Understanding and Dealing with the Japanese!* Singapore: Tuttle.

Everett, D. L. (2005). Cultural constraints on grammar and cognition in Pirahã: Another look at the design features of human language. *Current Anthropology, 46*(4): 621–646.

Fosse, M. J., Fosse, R., Hobson, J. A., & Stickgold, R. J. (2003). Dreaming and episodic memory: a functional dissociation? *Journal of Cognitive Neuroscience, 15*(1): 1–9.

Foulkes, W. D. (1962). Dream reports from different stages of sleep. *Journal of Abnormal Psychology & Social Psychology, 65*: 14–25.

Frank, R. (1969). *The Americans*. New York: HarperCollins.

Freud, S. (1900a). *The Interpretation of Dreams. S. E., 4–5*. London: Hogarth.

Freud, S. (1901b). *The Psychopathology of Everyday Life. S. E., 6*. London: Hogarth.

Goldberg, D. P., Oldehinkel, T., & Ormel, J. (1998). Why GHQ threshold varies from one place to another. *Psychological Medicine, 28*(4): 915–921.

Gomez, A. (interviewer) & Magritte, R. (nterviewee) (1948). *Radio Suisse Romande* [interview transcript]. Retrieved September 2016 from This is Not a Painter. *Harper's Magazine*: http://harpers.org/archive/2016/09/this-is-not-a-painter/

Greer, G. (1979). *The Obstacle Race: The Fortunes of Women Painters and Their Work*. New York: Farrar, Straus & Giroux.

Gross, J. (2009). *Handbook of Emotion Regulation*. New York: Guilford Press.

Hassin, R., Uleman, J., & Bargh, J. (2005). *The New Unconscious*. New York: Oxford University Press.

Herder, J. G. (1827). *Treatise upon the Origin of Language. Translated from the German*. London: Longman, Rees, Orme, Brown & Green.

Hill, C. E., & Knox, S. (2010). The use of dreams in modern psychotherapy. *International Review of Neurobiology, 92*: 291–317.

Hobson, J. A. (2009). REM sleep and dreaming: Towards a theory of protoconsciousness. *Nature Reviews Neuroscience, 10*(11): 803–813.

Hobson, J. A., & McCarley, R. W. (1977). The brain as a dream state generator: an activation-synthesis hypothesis of the dream process. *American Journal of Psychiatry, 134*(12): 1335–1348.

Huemer, J., Shaw, R. J., Prunas, A., Hall, R., Gross, J., & Steiner, H. (2015). Adolescent defense style as correlate of problem behavior. *Zeitschrift fur Kinder-und Jugendpsychiatrie und Psychotherapie, 43*(5): 345–350.

Hugo, V. (1874). *Quatre-vingt-treize*. Paris: M. Lévy frères.

Johnston, W. M. (1972). *The Austrian Mind: An Intellectual and Social History, 1848–1938*. Berkeley, CA: University of California Press.

Jouvet, M., & Jouvet, D. (1963). A study of the neurophysiological mechanisms of dreaming. *Electroencephalography and Clinical Neurophysiology*, Supplement 24: 133–157.

Kandel, E. R. (2012). *The Age of Insight: The Quest to Understand the Unconscious in Art, Mind, and Brain, from Vienna 1900 to the Present*. New York: Random House.

Khanzode, L., Kraemer, H., Saxena, K., Chang, K., & Steiner, H. (2006). Efficacy profiles of psychopharmacology: Divalproex sodium in conduct disorder. *Child Psychiatry and Human Development, 37*(1): 55–64.

Koch, C. (2012). Consciousness does not reside here. *Scientific American Mind, 23*(1): 20–21.

Kris, A. O. (2011). *Free Association: Method and Process, 2nd Edition*. London: Karnac.

Lakoff, G. (1993). How metaphor structures dreams: The theory of conceptual metaphor applied to dream analysis. *Dreaming, 3*(2): 77–98.

LeDoux, J. E. (2000). Emotion circuits in the brain. *Annual Review of Neuroscience, 23*: 155–184.

LeDoux, J. E. (2003). The emotional brain, fear, and the amygdala. *Cellular and Molecular Neurobiology, 23*(4–5): 727–738.

McCrae, R. R., & Costa, P. T. (2008). The five-factor theory of personality. In: O. P. John, R. W. Robins, & L. A. Pervin (Eds.), *Handbook of Personality. 3rd Edition: Theory and Research*. New York: Guilford Press.

McNamara, A. (2011). Can we measure memes? *Frontiers in Evolutionary Neuroscience, 3*(1): 1–7.

Mergenthaler, E., & Bucci, W. (1999). Linking verbal and nonverbal representations: Computer analysis of referential activity. *British Journal of Medical Psychology, 72*: 339–354.

Merton, T. (1955). *No Man Is an Island*. New York: Houghton Mifflin Harcourt.

Nelson, K. L., Bein, E., Ryst, E., Huemer, J., & Steiner, H. (2009). Listening for avoidance: Narrative form and defensiveness in adolescent memories. *Child Psychiatry and Human Development, 40*(4): 561–573.

Nelson, K. L., Moskovitz, D. J., & Steiner, H. (2008). Narration and vividness as measures of event-specificity in autobiographical memory. *Discourse Processes, 45*: 195–209.

Oudiette, D., Dealberto, M. J., Uguccioni, G., Golmard, J. L., Merino-Andreu, M., Tafti, M., Garma, L., Schwartz, S., & Arnulf, I. (2012). Dreaming without REM sleep. *Consciousness and Cognition, 21*(3): 1129–1140.

Ozment, S. (2004). *A Mighty Fortress: A New History of the German People*. New York: HarperCollins.

Rechtschaffen, A. (1971). The control of sleep. In: W. A. Hunt (Ed.), *Human Behavior and Its Control* (pp. 75–92). Cambridge, MA: Schenkman.

Ricoeur, P. (1970). *Freud and Philosophy. An Essay on Interpretation*. New Haven, CT: Yale University Press.

Rilke, R. M. (1997). *Rilke's Book of Hours: Love Poems to God (8th ed.)*. A. Barrows & J. Macy (Trans.). New York City: Riverhead.

Schachter, S., & Singer, J. E. (1962). Cognitive, social, and physiological determinants of emotional state. *Psychological Review, 69*: 379–399.

Shedler, J. (2010). The efficacy of psychodynamic psychotherapy. *American Psychologist, 65*(2): 98–109.

Siegel, J. M. (2011). REM sleep: A biological and psychological paradox. *Sleep Medicine Reviews, 15*(3): 139–142.

Solms, M. (1995). New findings on the neurological organization of dreaming: Implications for psychoanalysis. *Psychoanalytic Quarterly, 64*(1): 43–67.

Solms, M., & Turnbull, O. (2002). *The Brain and the Inner World: An Introduction to the Neuroscience of Subjective Experience*. New York: Other Press.

Steiner, H. (1977). Freud against himself. *Perspectives in Biology and Medicine, 20*(4): 510–527.

Steiner, H. (Ed.). (2011). *Handbook of Developmental Psychiatry*. Singapore: World Scientific Publishing.

Steiner, H. (2012). Laudatio for Irvin David Yalom, MD. *Z. f. Individualpsychol., 37*: 293–304.

Steiner, H., Araujo, K. B., & Koopman, C. (2001). The response evaluation measure (REM-71): A new instrument for the measurement of defenses in adults and adolescents. *American Journal of Psychiatry, 158*(3): 467–473.

Steiner, H. (Ed.) with Hall, R. (2015). *Treating Adolescents (2nd Edition)*. Westford, MA: Wiley.

Stickgold, R. (2005). Sleep-dependent memory consolidation. *Nature, 437*(7063): 1272–1278.

Stickgold, R., & Ellenbogen, J. (2008). Quiet! Sleeping brain at work. During slumber, our brain engages in data analysis, from strengthening memories to solving problems. *Scientific American Mind, 19*(4): 22–29.

Strawson, G. (2016, May 16). Consciousness isn't a mystery. It's matter. *The New York Times*. Retrieved from http://www.nytimes.com/2016/05/16/opinion/consciousness-isnt-a-mystery-its-matter.html?_r=0

Suzuki, H., Uchiyama, M., Tagaya, H., Ozaki, A., Kuriyama, K., Aritake, S., Shibui, K., Tan, X., Kamei, Y., & Kuga, R. (2004). Dreaming during non-rapid eye movement sleep in the absence of prior rapid eye movement sleep. *Sleep, 27*(8): 1486–1490.

Vieweg, B. W., & Hedlund, J. L. (1983). The General Health Questionnaire (GHQ): A comprehensive review. *Journal of Operational Psychiatry, 14*(2): 74–81.

Wamsley, E. J., & Stickgold, R. (2010). Dreaming and offline memory processing. *Current Biology, 20*(23): 1010–1013.

Weinberger, D. A., & Schwartz, G. E. (1990). Distress and restraint as superordinate dimensions of self-reported adjustment: A typological perspective. *Journal of Personality, 58*(2): 381–417.

Welch, F. S., Winters, R., & Ross, K. (2009). *Tea with Elisabeth: Tributes to Hospice Pioneer Dr. Elisabeth Kübler-Ross*. Naples, FL: Quality of Life Publishing.

Widom, C. S. (1989). The cycle of violence. *Science, 244*(4901): 160–166.

Wittgenstein, L. (1922). *Tractatus Logico-Philosophicus (TLP)*. C. K. Ogden (Trans.). London: Routledge & Kegan Paul. Originally published as Logisch-Philosophische Abhandlung in *Annalen der Naturphilosophische, XIV*(3/4), 1921.

Wolfe, T. (August 2016). The origins of speech. *Harper's Magazine*. Retrieved from http://harpers.org/archive/2016/08/the-origins-of-speech/

Zhang, J. (2005). Continual-activation theory of dreaming. *Dynamical Psychology*. Retrieved from http://www.goertzel.org/dynapsyc/2005/ZhangDreams.htm

INDEX

For Product Safety Concerns and Information please contact our EU representative GPSR@taylorandfrancis.com
Taylor & Francis Verlag GmbH, Kaufingerstraße 24, 80331 München, Germany

www.ingramcontent.com/pod-product-compliance
Ingram Content Group UK Ltd.
Pitfield, Milton Keynes, MK11 3LW, UK
UKHW022025061126
477531UK00002B/28

* 9 7 8 0 3 6 7 3 2 9 9 9 0 *